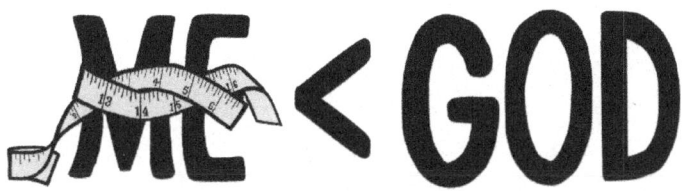

90 Days to Less of Me & More of You, God

A Weight Loss Devotional & Journal
Journaling Your Journey with God

Leslie Baldwin

Unless otherwise noted, all Scripture quotations and Biblical references are retrieved from https://www.biblegateway.com.

Copyright © 2018 by Leslie Baldwin

All rights reserved. In accordance with the U.S. Copyright Act of 1976, the scanning, uploading, and electronic sharing of any part of this book without the permission of the author is unlawful piracy and theft of the author's intellectual property. If you would like to use material from the book (other than for review purposes), prior written permission must be obtained by contacting the author at lesliertbsolutions@gmail.com. Thank you for the support of the author's rights.

ISBN: 9781728738468

Table of Contents

Introduction 6
Body Measurement Tracker Instructions 7
Day 1 – Poor Eating Habits? 14
Day 2 – No Grumbling 16
Day 3 – Self-Control 18
Day 4 – Unconditional Love 20
Day 5 – Focus on the Unseen 22
Day 6 – Doing What You Are Called to Do 24
Day 7 – God's Grace Needed 26
Day 8 – Let God Lead You 28
Day 9 – Be Strong & Very Courageous 30
Day 10 – Let God Be Seen Through Your Body 32
Day 11 – Stick Around and See What God Does 34
Day 12 – Be Thankful 36
Day 13 – Recover Your Life 38
Day 14 – Persistence & Progress, Not Perfection 40
Day 15 – Praise & Worship Through Weight Loss 42
Day 16 – This Won't Last Long 44
Day 17 – You Are Not Alone 46
Day 18 - Preparation 48
Day 19 – Don't Be Persuaded 50
Day 20 – Look Forward to Your "Why" 52
Day 21 – Finish the Work 54
Day 22 – Be Thankful 56
Day 23 – No Condemnation 58
Day 24 – I Want To Do What Is Right 60
Day 25 – He Knows All Your Needs 62
Day 26 – You Are Who You Are For a Reason 64
Day 27 – Nothing Can Separate You From His Love 66
Day 28 - Vantage Point 68
Day 29 – Let God Transform You 70
Day 30 – Let's Celebrate Together! 72
Day 31 – What You Need To Know When You Need To Know It 76

Day 32 – Ask, Using His Name 78
Day 33 – Not What You Did or How You Look 80
Day 34 – Every Detail of Your Life 82
Day 35 – Ask Questions 84
Day 36 – The Mud & The Mire 86
Day 37 – A Divine Process 88
Day 38 – See Yourself As He Sees You 90
Day 39 – More Than Anything 92
Day 40 – It Is Possible 94
Day 41 – In Spite of Temptation 96
Day 42 – Freedom to Choose 98
Day 43 – Benefits in This Life & The Life to Come 100
Day 44 – Wonderfully Complex 102
Day 45 - Day & Night 104
Day 46 – Diligent & Prepared 106
Day 47 – Made in His Image 108
Day 48 – He Knows Everything About You 110
Day 49 – In His Presence 112
Day 50 – Changing Your Thoughts & Actions 114
Day 51 – Don't Fall Into The Envy Trap 116
Day 52 – Heart, Mind, & Actions in Alignment 118
Day 53 – Disappointed, Discouraged, But Not Abandoned 120
Day 54 – Nothings Too Hard 122
Day 55 – Your Future 124
Day 56 – You Are Complete 126
Day 57 – Choice & Decision 128
Day 58 – A Gift From God 130
Day 59 – Free of Fear 132
Day 60 – In All Circumstances 134
Day 61 – By Teaching, We Learn 138
Day 62 – Non-Scale Victories 140
Day 63 – Peaceful Harvest of Right Living 142
Day 64 – Diligence Required 144
Day 65 – One Thing Will Never Change 146

Day 66 – You Have The Power 148
Day 67 – Day & Night 150
Day 68 – You Are Redeemed 152
Day 69 – Grace, Special Favor 154
Day 70 – Train Your Body 156
Day 71 – More Alike Than We Think 158
Day 72 – No Need to Compare Yourself 160
Day 73 – Healing The Brokenhearted 162
Day 74 – Hope & Encouragement 164
Day 75 – Who Told You That? 166
Day 76 – Nothing New Under The Sun 168
Day 77 – One Race 170
Day 78 - Promises 172
Day 79 – Advisers & Accountability 174
Day 80 – You Will Be Tempted 176
Day 81 – He Sees You 178
Day 82 – Infinitely More Than We Think 180
Day 83 – The Secret 182
Day 84 – Accept Yourself & Others 184
Day 85 – God Gives You The Power 186
Day 86 – Put On Your New Nature 188
Day 87 – We All Struggle at Times 190
Day 88 – Your Journey 192
Day 89 – Working Together For The Good 194
Day 90 – More Than Words…Well-Made Weapons 196
About the Author 199

Introduction

Losing weight is one of the most challenging things I've done. Primarily because I've lost and gained weight so many times in the past; I had gotten to the point that I was my heaviest, 307 pounds. I made a decision that I was going to lose 100 pounds and keep it off. Thus the real journey began. During my journey, after hitting a plateau for over five months, I realized that I was only relying on myself, not God.

No matter where you are in your journey, my prayer is that this devotional and journal will help you to have more of God and less of you.

How to use this devotional and journal:

As I've learned on my journey, mindfulness is so important because it helps you to think about what you are doing versus just mindlessly doing it. This devotional is set up to aid you with:

- Spending time with God each day, seeking Him, drawing closer to Him, through the scriptures shared daily, meditating on them, and praying the short daily prayer
- Journaling your thoughts. Research shows there are numerous benefits to journaling. I have found that journaling on a regular basis helps me to express my emotions in a natural, safe way, and to manage stress, which is a considerable factor in effectively losing weight and keeping it off.
- Tracking what you've eaten and how you are incorporating healthy habits daily, such as drinking water, and exercising.

I suggest that you only weigh yourself once a week and track your body measurements every other week. Remember that there are many successes on your journey outside of the scale, celebrate those also!

Body Measurement Tracker Instructions

Karl Pearson, an English mathematician, stated "Where performance is measured, performance improves. When performance is measured and reported back, the rate of improvement accelerates." Accelerate your progress by tracking it for the next 90 days. Instructions for taking body measurements:

- Weight – if possible use a digital scale that includes Body Fat %, Body Mass Index (BMI), Body Water %, and Bone Mass. Try to weigh on a weekly basis first thing in the morning before eating or drinking.

- Bust - Place the measuring tape across your nipples and measure around the largest part of your chest. Be sure to keep the tape parallel to the floor. How To Take Body Measurements | Sparkpeople. (n.d.). Retrieved from https://www.sparkpeople.com/resource/fitness_articles.asp?ID=1281

- Chest – Place the measuring tape just under your breasts/pecs and measure around the torso while keeping the tape parallel to the floor. How To Take Body Measurements | Sparkpeople. (n.d.). Retrieved from https://www.sparkpeople.com/resource/fitness_articles.asp?ID=1281

- Waist – Place the measuring tape about a 1/2 inch above your belly button (at the narrowest part of your waist) to measure around your torso. When measuring your waist, exhale and measure before inhaling again. How To Take Body Measurements | Sparkpeople. (n.d.). Retrieved from https://www.sparkpeople.com/resource/fitness_articles.asp?ID=1281

- Hips – Place the measuring tape across the widest part of your hips/buttocks and measure all the way around while keeping the tape parallel to the floor. How To Take Body Measurements | Sparkpeople. (n.d.). Retrieved from https://www.sparkpeople.com/resource/fitness_articles.asp?ID=1281

- Thighs – Measure around the largest part of each thigh. How To Take Accurate Body Measurements - Bloom. (n.d.). Retrieved from https://www.heybloom.com/2017/08/10/body-measurements/

- Calves – Measure around the largest part of each calf Body Measurement Tracking Chart - Thefitnessfocus.com. (n.d.). Retrieved from https://thefitnessfocus.com/fitness-tips/body-measurement-tracking-chart

- Upper Arm – Measure around the largest part of each arm (above the elbow).

- Forearm – Measure around the largest part of each arm (below the elbow).

- Neck – Measure around the largest part of the neck.

- Body Fat % - if your digital scale doesn't calculate it, use a calculator - https://www.verywellfit.com/how-to-use-body-fat-percentage-calculator-3858855

- Body Mass Index (BMI) – if your digital scale doesn't calculate it, the formula =Weight in Kilograms divided by Height (in meters) x Height (in meters) Beyond BMI: How To Calculate Body Fat Percentage ... (n.d.). Retrieved from https://food.ndtv.com/health/beyond-bmi-how-to-calculate-body-fat-percentage-122

- Body Water % - if your digital scale doesn't calculate it, use a calculator - https://www.omnicalculator.com/health/body-water

- Bone Mass – if your digital scale doesn't calculate it, use a calculator - http://en.fitnessyard.com/tools/body-mass-calculator

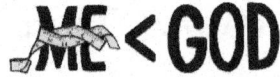

Body Measurement Tracker

Measurements:	Date: ___ / ___ / ___	___ / ___ / ___	___ / ___ / ___	___ / ___ / ___
Weight				
Bust				
Chest				
Waist				
Hips				
Thighs				
Calves				
Upper Arm				
Forearm				
Neck				
Body Fat %				
Body Mass Index (BMI)				
Body Water %				
Bone Mass				

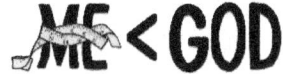

Body Measurement Tracker

Measurements:	Date: ___/___/___	___/___/___	___/___/___	___/___/___
Weight				
Bust				
Chest				
Waist				
Hips				
Thighs				
Calves				
Upper Arm				
Forearm				
Neck				
Body Fat %				
Body Mass Index (BMI)				
Body Water %				
Bone Mass				

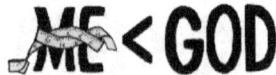

Body Measurement Tracker

Measurements:	Date: ___/___/___	___/___/___	___/___/___	___/___/___
Weight				
Bust				
Chest				
Waist				
Hips				
Thighs				
Calves				
Upper Arm				
Forearm				
Neck				
Body Fat %				
Body Mass Index (BMI)				
Body Water %				
Bone Mass				

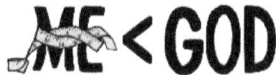

Body Measurement Tracker

Measurements:	Date: __/__/__	__/__/__	__/__/__	__/__/__
Weight				
Bust				
Chest				
Waist				
Hips				
Thighs				
Calves				
Upper Arm				
Forearm				
Neck				
Body Fat %				
Body Mass Index (BMI)				
Body Water %				
Bone Mass				

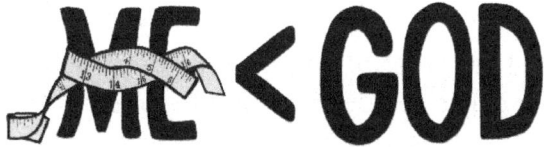

Voyage One

(voy•age — an account of a journey)

Day 1 – Poor Eating Habits?

So letting your sinful nature control your mind leads to death. But letting the Spirit control your mind leads to life and peace. Romans 8:6 NLT

Death really! It seems like the threat of death would be enough to keep anyone from doing anything that would cause it. But, if you are like me, and I suspect you are, that threat has not been enough to keep me from sabotaging my weight loss plan or goals.

Does God mean literal death or spiritual death? I think this is a common question. Literal death would mean the physical end of time here on earth. Spiritual death would mean separation from God. Though I believe, when I am physically no longer here on earth, I'll be in eternity with God; I've got some things I'd like to accomplish before then! So, both seem pretty bad to me.

So, how is it that the threat of either has not prohibited me from letting my sinful nature control my mind when it comes to poor eating habits? Is it because I don't see poor eating habits as a sin? Or is it because it is an addiction or a stronghold that is controlling my actions and behavior?

Whatever is keeping me from letting the Spirit control my mind, which would lead to life and peace, I want to change it.

Prayer: Lord, I let your Spirit control my mind, and I release my unhealthy desire for food.

Journal Your Journey: Have your eating habits become an addiction or stronghold in your life?

ME < GOD

Journal Your Journey:

Track Your Day - Date: _____/_____/_____

Breakfast	Snack	Lunch	Snack	Dinner	Snack

Water Intake:

Exercise:

Day 2 – No Grumbling

So whether you eat or drink, or whatever you do, do it all for the glory of God. And don't grumble as some of them did, and then were destroyed by the angel of death. 1 Corinthians 10:31, 10 NLT

Whenever I've been on restrictive eating plans, where I can't have certain things I've come to enjoy (like queso dip and chips) I get cranky, irritable, sad, and frustrated. I'll see other people (usually slimmer than I am) eat what they want to eat, and I am frustrated because why do they get to eat what they want and I don't!

I have compared myself to others most of my life, especially when it comes to my body image. I've often asked myself, "Am I the biggest person in the room?" This is torture to my self-esteem. (We'll deal with this topic later).

The reality is I can change my weight, and part of that process is eating a restrictive diet of fewer calories and a certain amount of macronutrients for a period of time. So, I've got to change my mindset when it comes to eating less and eating food that will help me achieve my goal.

A big part of that change is to not grumble or complain about what I am eating to reach my weight loss goal but instead, realize that whatever I eat or drink, do it all to the glory of God.

Prayer: God, I repent for grumbling and complaining about what I eat that is good for me, and I eat and drink that which is beneficial for my weight loss to your glory.

Journal Your Journey: How will you change your mindset about eating healthy?

ME < GOD

Journal Your Journey:

Track Your Day - Date: _____ / _____ / _____

Breakfast	Snack	Lunch	Snack	Dinner	Snack

Water Intake: ⊔ ⊔ ⊔ ⊔ ⊔ ⊔ ⊔

Exercise:

Day 3 – Self-Control

But the Holy Spirit produces this kind of fruit in our lives: love, joy, peace, patience, kindness, goodness, faithfulness, gentleness, and self-control. There is no law against these things! Galatians 5:22-23 NLT

Self-control, it can be elusive. Some days I feel like I am in control and disciplined; then at other times I am completely out of control and bingeing on sweets.

I was writing in my journal one day and asking God to give me discipline and self-control. The following day a good friend of ours, Pastor Terrance, ministered at church and during his message, he said: "Discipline is a self-imposed standard to achieve a desired goal." Self-imposed...you mean I control whether I am disciplined or not; it isn't something God does for me or to me! This message slapped me in my face, and I realized that all along, being in control of my eating and exercise is on me.

God loves us, and He wants us to have victory in every area of our lives. This includes winning the battle over our weight issues. We play a big part in achieving victory, and that is through discipline and self-control. It is a fruit of the Spirit, which means it comes as a result of allowing the Holy Spirit to lead and guide our lives, but it isn't automatic in that you can't just do nothing and still enjoy the results of that fruit. It is a self-imposed standard to achieve a desired goal.

Prayer: Lord, I welcome your Holy Spirit in my life and the manifestation of the fruit of your spirit. Right now Lord, I specifically pray for the manifestation of self-control. I realize that I play a part in having self-control and I am willing to do my part.

Journal Your Journey: Have you manifested self-control?

ME < GOD

Journal Your Journey:

Track Your Day - Date: _____/_____/_____

Breakfast	Snack	Lunch	Snack	Dinner	Snack

Water Intake:
🥛 🥛 🥛 🥛 🥛 🥛 🥛

Exercise:

Day 4 – Unconditional Love

Long ago the Lord said to Israel: "I have loved you, my people, with an everlasting love. With unfailing love I have drawn you to myself. Jeremiah 31:3 NLT

God loves you deeply! This is always a true statement, no matter what you do or don't do because it is unconditional love. He especially loves you when you don't love yourself. His love is what carries you through those times.

Most people look at me and believe that I have high self-esteem, but for most of my life I have been insecure and haven't loved myself. I know it was only God's love that got me through those years of self-loathing. Low self-esteem will still try to rear its ugly head in my life, and I have to remind myself that God loves me deeply!

Of course my issue with weight is a natural by-product of low self-esteem and as I've been on what I call my final weight loss journey (because my face is fixed like a flint and I am focused and have decided, I will not go around this mountain again), I am building my self-esteem with every pound lost.

There have been many weeks where I've lost nothing or have even gained instead of lost. I've been frustrated, disappointed, and discouraged. During those times, I reflect on how much I have lost, and I thank God for it.

Be encouraged my friend, if you are in a place of low self-esteem or are not seeing the progress you want, remember, God loves you deeply, and His love is everlasting, and it is not based on your performance, how you look, or whether you never lose another pound. He loves you just as you are, and you are beautiful in His eyes!

Prayer: God, thank you for loving me, especially when I didn't love myself. Thank you that as I learn to love myself, it is because I am trusting and loving you more and more and that it has nothing to do with how I look or how much I weigh because that doesn't matter to you and it shouldn't matter to me.

Journal Your Journey: Do you realize that God loves you deeply?

ME < GOD

Journal Your Journey:

___

Track Your Day - Date: _____/_____/_____

Breakfast	Snack	Lunch	Snack	Dinner	Snack

Water Intake:
⬜ ⬜ ⬜ ⬜ ⬜ ⬜

Exercise:

Day 5 – Focus on the Unseen

So we don't look at the troubles we can see now; rather, we fix our gaze on things that cannot be seen. For the things we see now will soon be gone, but the things we cannot see will last forever. 2 Corinthians 4:18 NLT

I have not reached my goal of losing 100 lbs and keeping it off. For almost a year now, I have been saying, writing, and believing I will lose 100 lbs and keep it off; yet it has not manifested. At the time of this writing, I've lost 43 pounds and kept it off.

I don't look at the troubles I see now (that I have 57 lbs to lose to reach my goal), rather I fix my gaze on how I will feel and look when I lose 100 pounds. I know this time, my weight loss will be permanent, and so it will last forever. This is called faith.

When I read one of the study notes on 2 Corinthians 4:18, it said that the contrast is not really on visible and invisible realities, but more about what is "already" and what is "not yet." Focus your attention on what has not yet happened (your goal weight) and believe that it will come to pass. Think about how you will feel and what it will mean to you when you reach your goal. The body you see now will soon be gone forever!

Prayer: God, help me to keep my eyes fixed on what is unseen: my ultimate weight loss goal. Help me to be thankful for what has already happened: the weight I have already lost.

Journal Your Journey: Write a statement in your journal, "I will lose X pounds and keep it off." How will you focus on what is "not yet"?

ME < GOD

Journal Your Journey:

Track Your Day - Date: _____/_____/_____

Breakfast	Snack	Lunch	Snack	Dinner	Snack

Water Intake: 🥛 🥛 🥛 🥛 🥛 🥛 🥛

Exercise:

Day 6 – Doing What You Are Called to Do

For we are God's masterpiece. He has created us anew in Christ Jesus, so we can do the good things he planned for us long ago. Ephesians 2:10 NLT

Has your weight kept you from doing things you desired to do? Being overweight has prevented me from doing several things I've desired to do. Recently two of my friends decided to go skydiving and extended the invitation to a group of us. Everyone in the group didn't have the desire to go, but I did! I was excited about it and agreed to join them. My friend provided the details and the instructions on how to go online to schedule it. I pulled up the website and was following the instructions to book our time slot, and something said, "Read through the FAQs first."

We were planning to do tandem jumping, which means you are physically connected to an experienced skydiver as you jump out of the plane together. The experienced skydiver handles the majority of the controls for you. The FAQs listed a recommended weight limit for tandem jumping and yes, you guessed it, I was over the weight limit.

If this had happened to me just a few years ago, I would have been embarrassed, devastated and would have been dishonest with my friend about why I couldn't go, when I had already agreed to go. Since I have decided I will lose 100 lbs and keep it off, I knew I'd get below the minimum weight requirement soon. I sent my friend a text message and told her that I couldn't go because of my weight and that once I got below the weight limit, I'd plan on going then. She immediately called me and was so excited for me and said she would be looking forward to celebrating with me and going again at that time.

Don't allow your weight to hinder you any longer from doing what you desire or what you believe God has called you to do. For we are God's masterpiece, He has created us anew in Christ Jesus so we can do the good things He planned for us long ago. Skydiving may not be the good thing He planned for you long ago (or me either for that matter)! But, you are His masterpiece, and He has a plan for you, and you have to be able to do what He has planned. Don't let your weight stop you; whatever the reason, physical limitations or self-imposed limitations.

Prayer: God, I want to do all that you have called me to do, and I know that my physical, mental and spiritual well being plays a part in what you've planned. Thank you that I will be at a healthy weight and that my weight will never deter me from doing what you've called me to do.

Journal Your Journey: What has your weight hindered you from doing that you desire to do?

ME < GOD

Journal Your Journey:

Track Your Day - Date: _____ / _____ / _____

Breakfast	Snack	Lunch	Snack	Dinner	Snack

Water Intake: ◯ ◯ ◯ ◯ ◯ ◯ ◯ ◯

Exercise:

Day 7 – God's Grace Needed

Each time he said, "My grace is all you need. My power works best in weakness." So now I am glad to boast about my weaknesses, so that the power of Christ can work through me. 2 Corinthians 12:9 NLT

As I was writing today's devotional, it felt forced, like it wasn't what God wanted me to share. I've been on a new eating plan for the last seven days. It is very specific; I eat five preportioned meals and one meal that I prepare of protein and vegetables. It has helped me with keeping it simple regarding what to eat.

The seventh day into the new eating plan was Father's Day, and I baked for my husband and my son (it was my son's first Father's Day!). My husband wanted a red velvet cake, and my son wanted a chocolate cake with chocolate frosting. For me, it can be challenging to stay away from sweets in general, so just imagine being the one baking. I had decided this would be a good test of my will power. I did well with the red velvet cake; baked, frosted, and nothing in my mouth!

As I was preparing to frost the chocolate cake, I realized that it was the first time I had made this cake from scratch and not from a box, and I thought what if it doesn't taste good. So, as I was piercing the cake with a fork (to let the frosting melt into the cake), a small piece of the cake was on the fork, and I took a tiny bit and put it in my mouth. Immediately, I felt guilt, regret, and disappointment.

I have felt this way before; perhaps you have too. I was reminded that God's grace is sufficient for me. Which means that although I ate something that wasn't a part of my eating plan, God's grace (His unmerited favor) frees me from guilt, regret, and disappointment and allows me to refocus and carry on immediately.

How do you receive His grace? God freely gives it to all who believe in Him. You ask Him for it and believe that you've received it. God says, His power works best in weakness. My weakness, eating a tiny piece of the cake, is when God's power works best if I allow it to work. In the past, I would have wallowed in my guilt, regret, and disappointment or ate even more since I had already messed up my eating plan. This time I remembered that His grace is all I need.

Prayer: God, thank you that your grace is all I need and that it is sufficient for every situation where I am weak.

Journal Your Journey: Have you or are you wallowing in guilt, regret, or disappointment?

ME < GOD

Journal Your Journey:

Track Your Day - Date: _____/_____/_____

Breakfast	Snack	Lunch	Snack	Dinner	Snack

Water Intake: ◯ ◯ ◯ ◯ ◯ ◯ ◯

Exercise:

Day 8 – Let God Lead You

We can make our plans, but the Lord determines our steps. Proverbs 16:9 NLT

My plan: I will lose 100 lbs and keep it off. I started this journey on July 13, 2017, and I thought by July 13, 2018, the weight would be off and I'd be living happily ever after 100 lbs lighter. It is June 18, 2018, almost a year from when I started and I am only down 46.5 lbs. I have fluctuated up and down in the era of my journey that I call the 260s for the past 5 months, and I finally feel like I am coming out of this decade of my weight loss journey!

Why God? Why hasn't my plan gone the way I thought it would? Why have I struggled in what feels like the same place for the past 5 months?

God said, "You were doing it in your strength." I realized He was right. It was my plan and my thoughts of when it should happen. I would have gotten the glory. But, that was not God's plan. He patiently waited for me to come to Him with my questions and my frustration. From that, He birthed the idea of this weight loss devotional and journal. I believe He will use this for His glory! God's plan is so much better than our plans. He doesn't tell us not to make plans, not to dream, or not to take action. He wants us to dream, plan, and take action; He just wants us to allow Him to lead and guide us through it. Trust that His plan for you is good and that it will give you hope and a future far more significant than you ever imagined!

Prayer: God, thank you for determining my steps in this weight loss journey and for leading and guiding me through it. I trust you, and I know that I will reach my goals. I will give you all of the glory.

Journal Your Journey: Who is leading your weight loss journey, you or God?

ME < GOD

Journal Your Journey:

Track Your Day - Date: _____/_____/_____

Breakfast	Snack	Lunch	Snack	Dinner	Snack

Water Intake:
▢ ▢ ▢ ▢ ▢ ▢ ▢

Exercise:

Day 9 – Be Strong & Very Courageous

No one will be able to stand against you as long as you live. For I will be with you as I was with Moses. I will not fail you or abandon you. Be strong and very courageous. Be careful to obey all the instructions Moses gave you. Do not deviate from them, turning either to the right or to the left. Then you will be successful in everything you do. Joshua 1:5,7 NLT

Talking openly about my weight challenges is difficult for me. It is not something I am doing in and of myself; it is definitely through the power and strength of God. I have been self-conscious and unhappy with my weight for so long that I had started to settle with being overweight.

Finally, I can see the light at the end of this weight loss tunnel. I still experience feelings of being afraid that I am going to fail and wanting to deviate from the plan I am on. Even though I know deviating from the plan will cause me to not be successful or reach my goal, the feeling to deviate pops up and lingers at times.

It takes strength and courage to stick with a plan and reach a goal, it will take even more strength and courage to not gain the weight back and maintain it. Sometimes you have to draw on that strength and courage around your family and friends when they try to sway you or encourage you to eat the things they are eating.

I'm sure you've heard some of the same things I've heard: you've got to live a little; one little piece has never hurt anyone, or you have to eat something. It can feel like you are the odd man out when you're sticking to your plan and no one around you is in that same place. Those are the times to remember that God is with you and that He will not fail you or abandon you. Be strong and very courageous.

Prayer: God, thank you for always being with me and helping me to be strong and courageous throughout this journey to lose weight and to keep it off.

Journal Your Journey: What does being strong and courageous look like for you?

ME < GOD

Journal Your Journey:

Track Your Day - Date: _____/_____/_____

Breakfast	Snack	Lunch	Snack	Dinner	Snack

Water Intake:

Exercise:

Day 10 – Let God Be Seen Through Your Body

Or didn't you realize that your body is a sacred place, the place of the Holy Spirit? Don't you see that you can't live however you please, squandering what God paid such a high price for? The physical part of you is not some piece of property belonging to the spiritual part of you. God owns the whole works. So let people see God in and through your body. 1 Corinthians 6:19-20 MSG

It is interesting how people categorize sin: murder, adultery, or stealing as big sins; whereas gossip, overindulgence, or little white lies are small sins. Sin is sin; it doesn't matter what our society says about it. What matters, is what God says about it.

Even though in this passage of scripture, God is talking about sexual sin and what it does to your body and your soul, it can be easily applied to what we do to our bodies when we overeat, don't exercise, or don't take care of the body God has given us to steward.

Many of us who struggle with food, may not struggle with sex or promiscuity and yet may look at people who do struggle with promiscuity, harsher than we look at ourselves. I'm here to tell you, my friend, it is no different. Both are sins against the body. That same feeling of regret, loneliness, or emptiness is felt when we overeat or have sex without commitment, covenant, and intimacy. God isn't pleased with either.

God forgives us of our sins and gives us mercy and grace. Remember we are all struggling with something; be gracious to others and yourself. As today's scripture states, let people see God in and through your body.

Prayer: God, I desire for people to see you in and through my body. Help me to be a good steward over this body that you have given me. Help me to receive your mercy and grace and extend that to others.

Journal Your Journey: Are you being a good steward over your body?

ME < GOD

Journal Your Journey:

Track Your Day - Date: _____/_____/_____

Breakfast	Snack	Lunch	Snack	Dinner	Snack

Water Intake: ⬭ ⬭ ⬭ ⬭ ⬭ ⬭ ⬭

Exercise:

Day 11 – Stick Around and See What God Does

But me, I'm not giving up. I'm sticking around to see what God will do. I'm waiting for God to make things right. I'm counting on God to listen to me. Micah 7:7 MSG

A good friend of mine who is attending Rhema Bible College sent me some books and a bracelet. The bracelet read - "I CANNOT BE DEFEATED AND I WILL NOT QUIT." With God on my side, I really can't be defeated. That is such a comforting feeling to know that ultimately I win with God.

When it comes to the "I will not quit" part... that requires me making a decision and is not about the surety of God. But, I have determined, that I'm not giving up. I am going to reach my goal to lose 100 lbs and keep it off. What is your goal? Have you finally decided that no matter what, you are going to achieve your goal?

I am confident that if I do the things I have control over, consistently eating right and exercising, that I'll get the results I want. Now from my experience, this is easier said than done, but I am going to do my part! I am sticking around to see what God will do, and I know that God will make it right.

Prayer: I will not quit, God. Thank you that I can be confident about this journey because you are with me, which means I cannot be defeated.

Journal Your Journey: Have you finally decided that no matter what, you are going to achieve your goal?

ME < GOD

Journal Your Journey:

Track Your Day - Date: _____/_____/_____

Breakfast	Snack	Lunch	Snack	Dinner	Snack

Water Intake:

Exercise:

Day 12 – Be Thankful

I will offer you a sacrifice of thanksgiving and call on the name of the Lord. Psalm 116:17 NLT

It is easy to only see how far you have to go to reach your goal, or how much you have to do to get there. You can easily fall into a place of being frustrated, feeling self-pity, and thinking that you are the only one who has to deal with "this."

When you find yourself in that place, begin to thank God for everything. Thankfulness will awaken you to God's presence, and thanksgiving will overshadow those feelings. It will seem foreign at first to be saying "thank you" in the midst of feeling frustrated or troubled, but try it and see how you begin to feel.

Be thankful for how far you have come on your weight loss journey. Be thankful that you're not where you use to be. Be thankful for the ability to move and exercise. Be thankful for the support from family, friends, or coaches. Be thankful that God gives you the ability to choose to be healthy and to live in a place where you have the freedom to do so. Thank Him for everything and call on His name.

Prayer: God, thank you for everything.

Journal Your Journey: What are you thankful for about your weight loss journey?

ME < GOD

Journal Your Journey:

Track Your Day - Date: _____/_____/_____

Breakfast	Snack	Lunch	Snack	Dinner	Snack

Water Intake:
☐ ☐ ☐ ☐ ☐ ☐ ☐ ☐

Exercise:

Day 13 – Recover Your Life

"Are you tired? Worn out? Burned out on religion? Come to me. Get away with me and you'll recover your life. I'll show you how to take a real rest. Walk with me and work with me—watch how I do it. Learn the unforced rhythms of grace. I won't lay anything heavy or ill-fitting on you. Keep company with me and you'll learn to live freely and lightly." Matthew 11:28 - 30 MSG

I am not a funny person. My husband is, and he makes me laugh most of the time. I tend to be more serious and reserved, and that can be heavy. I can laugh at myself and often do. I'll do things, and they are just ditzy, and I have to laugh even when no one else is with me to laugh.

But, living freely and lightly is hard to do when you are worried about something important to you, like your weight. I have been worried about my weight for the majority of my life, so it is a burden that I have carried. I am tired, fed up and worn out by losing weight and gaining it back; then struggling to lose it again. It is a forced rhythm of sadness, frustration, and pain.

God says come to me; get away with me, and you'll recover your life...learn the unforced rhythm of grace; and that He won't lay anything heavy or ill-fitting on us. God can lighten the heavy burden of worrying about your weight,

Prayer: God, thank you for showing me how to live lightly and freely. I will no longer allow fear about my weight to be forefront in my mind. Instead, I choose to come with you and recover my life.

Journal Your Journey: Have you struggled to lose weight and allowed it to mentally weigh you down?

ME < GOD

Journal Your Journey:

Track Your Day - Date: _____/_____/_____

Breakfast	Snack	Lunch	Snack	Dinner	Snack

Water Intake:

Exercise:

Day 14 – Persistence & Progress, Not Perfection

Do you see what this means—all these pioneers who blazed the way, all these veterans cheering us on? It means we'd better get on with it. Strip down, start running—and never quit! No extra spiritual fat, no parasitic sins. Keep your eyes on Jesus, who both began and finished this race we're in. Study how he did it. Because he never lost sight of where he was headed—that exhilarating finish in and with God—he could put up with anything along the way: Cross, shame, whatever. And now he's there , in the place of honor, right alongside God. When you find yourselves flagging in your faith, go over that story again, item by item, that long litany of hostility he plowed through. That will shoot adrenaline into your souls!
Hebrews 12:1-3 MSG

Weight loss is an equal opportunity issue, meaning it doesn't matter whether you are black or white, tall or short, rich or poor, it is something you have to do for yourself, and no one else can do it for you. The good news: if others have done it (successfully lost weight and kept it off), you can too!

You don't have to do everything it takes to lose weight perfectly; because frankly, none of us are perfect, only God is perfect. So you will not do anything perfectly anyway. What you can strive for is persistence which will result in progress.

Like Jesus, never lose sight of where you are headed so you can finish this weight loss journey. When the burden seems heavy, when you don't have people supporting you, when no one understands your struggle, or people doubt you'll succeed, remember if others have done it, you can too. Remember persistence and progress, not perfection.

Persistence & Progress Ø Perfection

Prayer: God, help me to continue to be persistent in this journey to lose weight. Thank you for your ultimate example of what you endured to save me.

Journal Your Journey: *Do you find yourself striving to be perfect instead of persistent?*

ME < GOD

Journal Your Journey:

Track Your Day - Date: _____/_____/_____

Breakfast	Snack	Lunch	Snack	Dinner	Snack

Water Intake: ☐ ☐ ☐ ☐ ☐ ☐ ☐

Exercise:

Day 15 – Praise & Worship Through Weight Loss

This is the day the Lord has made. We will rejoice and be glad in it. Psalm 118:24 NLT

You know that feeling you get when you get on the scale and you've lost weight: the joy, excitement, and pleasure of seeing the fruits of your efforts; that feeling is the same feeling that we should have as we worship and praise God daily.

Worship and praise are different even though we often use them interchangeably. It doesn't take music to worship and praise God, though you can include it if you desire. Worship, although you can do it publicly, is something you can do that no one but you and God knows you are doing. It is intimate, personal, and a direct conversation between you and God.

Praise is an outward expression where you show God and others how good He is. In a class we taught at church about praise and worship, it said praise means to make a show, to boast, to be clamorously foolish. That sounds like fun to me! Praise is also an opportunity to make your flesh submit to your spirit especially when you may not feel like it.

Daily we can show others how good God is through our lives and this includes through our weight loss, healthy habits, and lifestyle.

Prayer: God I praise you, I thank you for this day, and the ability to rejoice and show others your goodness through my life.

Journal Your Journey: How can you praise and worship God through your weight loss?

ME < GOD

Journal Your Journey:

Track Your Day - Date: _____/_____/_____

Breakfast	Snack	Lunch	Snack	Dinner	Snack

Water Intake:
◯ ◯ ◯ ◯ ◯ ◯ ◯

Exercise:

Day 16 – This Won't Last Long

For our present troubles are small and won't last very long. Yet they produce for us a glory that vastly outweighs them and will last forever! 2 Corinthians 4:17 NLT

Your journey may not be like mine. Mine has been going on since I was in high school trying to lose weight. Although in the realm of my world it seems like a long time, it isn't a long time in the realm of the spirit because God is timeless.

It gives me hope to know that this present situation won't last very long, but will produce results that far outweigh the journey. Although some days it seems hard to do the things that I know I should do, I do them and remind myself...this won't last long. When my flesh is weak, and I don't want to exercise...this won't last long. When I am craving something sweet and I want to eat a whole bag of Oreos...this won't last long. As I focus on doing the things that bring about the health and results I want, by the grace of God my desires change.

So, keep going my friend, taking it one day and one step at a time knowing...this won't last long.

Prayer: God, thank you for this season in my life and for reminding me that it won't last long.

Journal Your Journey: Have you settled in your spirit that this won't last long?

ME < GOD

Journal Your Journey:

___

Track Your Day - Date: _____/_____/_____

Breakfast	Snack	Lunch	Snack	Dinner	Snack

Water Intake:
◯ ◯ ◯ ◯ ◯ ◯ ◯

Exercise:

Day 17 – You Are Not Alone

Don't be afraid, for I am with you. Don't be discouraged, for I am your God. I will strengthen you and help you. I will hold you up with my victorious right hand. Isaiah 41:10 NLT

Do you ever feel like you are on this journey alone? I do, and at times I am sad about it, and I am afraid of failing. Getting support from family, friends, or other like-minded people on your journey is key to your success.

The amazing thing is that God is always with you! He is there when all of your support from others is there, and He is there when there is no one else you can rely on. So when you feel discouraged, turn to God by talking to Him, journaling your thoughts, or sitting quietly in His presence.

God will hold you up with His victorious right-hand means that He is strong, faithful, and can be relied on to help you be victorious in every situation. This promise means we do not have to fear failure when we rely on God.

Prayer: I will not be afraid of failure because you, God, are with me and will help me be victorious.

Journal Your Journey: Do you realize that you are not alone?

ME < GOD

Journal Your Journey:

Track Your Day - Date: _____/_____/_____

Breakfast	Snack	Lunch	Snack	Dinner	Snack

Water Intake: ◻ ◻ ◻ ◻ ◻ ◻ ◻

Exercise:

Day 18 - Preparation

This all happened on Friday, the day of preparation, the day before the Sabbath. As evening approached, Mark 15:42 NLT

In the past, because I confess and believe that I have changed, I've not usually been on time and have been somewhat of a procrastinator. To me, it just felt unnatural being early to an event. If it started at 9:00 and I showed up at 8:45, I would always feel like I was inconveniencing the person or being rude by being early when they were expecting me at 9:00. If it was an event I was going to, I thought about what I would do for 15 minutes before the event started. Conversely, I didn't feel like it was rude to be late and show up after 9:00. (Don't judge me!)

Of course, this perspective of time management spilled over into other areas of my life such as my ability to plan effectively. One area of planning that is important when working on losing weight is meal prep. Knowing what you're going to eat and when is essential to your success. I still have not mastered this, but I enlisted the help of a plan that makes it virtually foolproof, like weight loss for dummies.

It's like that old saying "prior preparation relieves future frustration." Find what works for you, but know that to have sustained results, you've got to prepare ahead of time.

Today's passage of scripture is about planning for Jesus' burial, which for us as Believers marked the beginning of the most important day: the day He rose from the grave! There was a day full of preparation. Preparation is vital in so many areas of our lives, including in our weight loss journey.

Prayer: God, thank you for giving us the best example of the importance of preparation and for growing this habit and skill of effectively preparing in our lives.

Journal Your Journey: Are you preparing what you need to be successful on your weight loss journey?

ME < GOD

Journal Your Journey:

Track Your Day - Date: _____/_____/_____

Breakfast	Snack	Lunch	Snack	Dinner	Snack

Water Intake:
◯ ◯ ◯ ◯ ◯ ◯ ◯

Exercise:

Day 19 – Don't Be Persuaded

When it was clear that we couldn't persuade him, we gave up and said, "The Lord's will be done." Acts 21:14 NLT

I recently attended a Family Reunion. These types of events are special and fun because you get to see family and friends you haven't seen or spent time with in a while; however, they can sabotage your weight loss goals.

You want to be able to enjoy yourself and not feel guilty about what you eat because that is not living a life of freedom. However, you also don't want to set yourself back from what you've been working towards. A great way to find balance is to plan what you will eat and take with you the food options that will allow you to eat and enjoy with the rest of the family without sabotaging your plan.

Of course, there will be some people who will think you are extreme; that it doesn't take all of that; that you can be off plan for a few days. Don't allow anyone else to persuade you or determine what is best for you or make you feel bad for doing what is best for you. Stand firm on what you believe and what you are led to do.

Prayer: God, thank you for my conviction to stand firm and that I will not be persuaded by others who don't see or agree with my actions to reach my goals.

Journal Your Journey: Have you allowed yourself to be persuaded by others when it comes to your weight loss journey?

ME < GOD

Journal Your Journey:

Track Your Day - Date: _____/_____/_____

Breakfast	Snack	Lunch	Snack	Dinner	Snack

Water Intake:

Exercise:

Day 20 – Look Forward to Your "Why"

No, dear brothers and sisters, I have not achieved it, but I focus on this one thing: Forgetting the past and looking forward to what lies ahead, Philippians 3:13 NLT

It can be frustrating and disappointing when people don't notice or comment about your weight loss. Although you are not losing weight for that purpose, it is nice to get that bit of encouragement when someone sees the results of your efforts and tells you so.

The reality is whether anyone ever acknowledges it or not, you have to lose the weight and get healthy because you desire it and you are doing it for your big "why" and no one else. What is your "why"? I have several: I want to be able to walk into any store and buy clothes if I desire; I want to be healthy and fit; I want to feel good about my body; I want to skydive.

Experts say knowing and remembering your "why" is essential during those times that you may be struggling with staying focused and moving forward. I think it is also essential because you are clear about why you are heading in the direction you are heading while on your journey.

Prayer: God, let me be focused and clear regarding why I am on this journey and to never look back or waiver from it.

Journal Your Journey: What is your "Why"?

ME < GOD

Journal Your Journey:

Track Your Day - Date: _____/_____/_____

Breakfast	Snack	Lunch	Snack	Dinner	Snack

Water Intake: ◯ ◯ ◯ ◯ ◯ ◯ ◯

Exercise:

Day 21 – Finish the Work

But my life is worth nothing to me unless I use it for finishing the work assigned me by the Lord Jesus—the work of telling others the Good News about the wonderful grace of God. Acts 20:24 NLT

You are the common denominator in every situation that involves you. This means if you are a part of the situation you have a choice on how you react. This can be a hard fact to face because it doesn't allow you any room to blame others for the things that happen in your life. You always have the opportunity to choose your response.

Whether you ever lose weight or not, you are still you. You are still a beloved child of God; created and made in His image; able to do all things through His strength; fearfully and wonderfully made; a conqueror; and an overcomer.

Your weight doesn't stop you from doing what He has called you to do. However, it might make it easier to do what He has called you to do, with less weight on your body. But trust me, my friend, if you yield to God and allow Him to use you, lead and guide you; you can do anything.

Prayer: God, I will not let my weight stop me from doing what you've called me to do. I am yours. Use me how you see fit, God.

Journal Your Journey: Are you finishing the work assigned to you by God?

ME < GOD

Journal Your Journey:

Track Your Day - Date: _____/_____/_____

Breakfast	Snack	Lunch	Snack	Dinner	Snack

Water Intake:
☐ ☐ ☐ ☐ ☐ ☐ ☐

Exercise:

Day 22 – Be Thankful

Enter his gates with thanksgiving; go into his courts with praise. Give thanks to him and praise his name. Psalm 100:4 NLT

In my journey to lose 100 pounds, I stalled out around 40 pounds lost and stayed there for over 5 months. As of this writing, it has been almost a year since I started and I am officially down 52 pounds. As I calculated how many pounds that was in 12 months, it averaged out to 4.33 pounds per month. Although I am disappointed that I didn't lose 100 pounds in a year, I am thankful for losing 52.

Yesterday, I was talking with a friend that started a weight loss plan, and she too has a significant amount of weight to lose. She had lost 5 pounds during her first week on her plan. I asked, "It feels great, doesn't it?" She said, "It's okay." I realized that for many of us, it is easy to focus on what didn't happen versus being grateful for what did happen. When the scale doesn't move the way we hope, we can get down on ourselves and start to think it isn't working or not working as fast as we would like.

God desires for us to thank Him in every situation, good or bad. Our posture of thanksgiving is what brings us into His presence, which helps us to deal with any situation. Thank Him when you lose and thank Him when you don't. Be thankful.

Prayer: Thank you, God, for my weight lost and thank you for being with me even when the scale doesn't move. I trust you, God, and won't allow disappointment to keep me from thanking you.

Journal Your Journey: Write about what you are thankful for on this weight loss journey.

ME < GOD

Journal Your Journey:

Track Your Day - Date: _____/_____/_____

Breakfast	Snack	Lunch	Snack	Dinner	Snack

Water Intake:
⊔ ⊔ ⊔ ⊔ ⊔ ⊔ ⊔

Exercise:

Day 23 – No Condemnation

So now there is no condemnation for those who belong to Christ Jesus. Romans 8:1 NLT

Do you ever look at your body and wonder, how did I get here? Why have I allowed myself to be overweight? Why have I not lost this weight? I have, and waves of guilt, shame, and pain come, and they paralyze me from taking action.

The enemy will try to bombard your mind with these types of thoughts. Thoughts that keep you locked in a place of defeat and hopelessness. But, God came that we might have freedom. Freedom from these gripping thoughts; freedom from behaviors that have kept us in bondage; freedom from habits that have perpetuated our situations.

Once you accept Christ as your Lord and Savior, He releases us from the chains that bind us. We have to accept it and believe it. There is now no condemnation to those who belong to Him, meaning, anything you've done or will do, you stand before God perfect in His sight. Live in that freedom.

Prayer: God, thank you for revealing to me that feelings of guilt and shame are a lie and that in your sight I am perfect and free.

Journal Your Journey: Have you wondered how you got here, as in needing to lose weight?

ME < GOD

Journal Your Journey:

Track Your Day - Date: _____/_____/_____

Breakfast	Snack	Lunch	Snack	Dinner	Snack

Water Intake:

Exercise:

Day 24 – I Want To Do What Is Right

I have discovered this principle of life—that when I want to do what is right, I inevitably do what is wrong. I love God's law with all my heart. But there is another power within me that is at war with my mind. This power makes me a slave to the sin that is still within me. Oh, what a miserable person I am! Who will free me from this life that is dominated by sin and death? Thank God! The answer is in Jesus Christ our Lord. So you see how it is: In my mind I really want to obey God's law, but because of my sinful nature I am a slave to sin. Romans 7:21-25 NLT

I have been struggling with snacking on walnuts throughout the day. I know that eating too many will hinder my weight loss and could cause me to gain weight. Every day I tell myself that I won't eat any and inevitably I end up with a handful multiple times throughout the day. So, then I tell myself, I won't eat any tomorrow! The struggle is real! Do you have a similar type of struggle?

Take comfort in knowing we are not alone. All of us, just like Paul, the author of the book of Romans, struggle with something. Wanting to do what is right, like not eating that which we know will keep us from losing weight, but inevitably find ourselves doing the opposite. During those times we realize, like Paul, what miserable people we are for giving in to our desires.

But, thanks be to God who frees us from sin. Our faith and belief in Christ allow us to live by the Spirit and to set our minds on what the Spirit desires instead of what the flesh desires. It is an active process of calling on the Spirit during those moments and being dominated by the Spirit. You may not succeed at it every time those moments come, but the more you call on the Holy Spirit to help you during those times, the easier it will become to resist.

Prayer: God, I call on your Holy Spirit to dominate my mind and to free me from the desires of my flesh.

Journal Your Journey: What have you been struggling with on your weight loss journey?

ME < GOD

Journal Your Journey:

Track Your Day - Date: _____/_____/_____

Breakfast	Snack	Lunch	Snack	Dinner	Snack

Water Intake: ▢ ▢ ▢ ▢ ▢ ▢ ▢

Exercise:

Day 25 – He Knows All Your Needs

"So don't worry about these things, saying, 'What will we eat? What will we drink? What will we wear?' These things dominate the thoughts of unbelievers, but your heavenly Father already knows all your needs. Seek the Kingdom of God above all else, and live righteously, and he will give you everything you need. Matthew 6:31-33 NLT

I have many size clothes in my closet, from my largest at size 24 down to size 14. As I've lost and gained weight over the years, it is a juggling act with my wardrobe. I am not really sure when to buy new clothes for the size I am at, knowing I will lose more weight. But, I also don't want to wear larger sizes, because it makes me feel like I haven't accomplished much. I enjoy the sense of accomplishment when I feel and look good in smaller sizes.

However, I start to worry about wasting money on buying more clothes when I could be using that money for other things. I worry about the possibility of gaining the weight back after I've given away my larger size clothes and the personal defeat of having to go repurchase larger sizes. Have you experienced this crazy cycle?

When I am in this place, I remember God's word, that He already knows my needs. He already knows what I am going to do before I do it. He has always provided whatever I've needed, and I recognize and acknowledge how blessed I am, in spite of senselessly worrying.

I start to refocus on what is really important: seeking the Kingdom of God. This includes sharing our surplus with those who need it, by giving away the clothes I can no longer wear, all sizes, knowing it will bless others. As the Zondervan NIV study Bible indicates, when God's people give of their surplus to others, "all these things" (food, drink, clothing) will be given to them, and this is how the poor receive what they need. Shift your focus from yourself and give to others out of your surplus.

Prayer: God, thank you that you know all of my needs and the needs of others. I thank you that you trust me to be obedient to give out of my surplus to help meet the needs of other believers.

Journal Your Journey: Have you gotten rid of your larger size clothing? If not, why?

ME < GOD

Journal Your Journey:

Track Your Day - Date: _____ / _____ / _____

Breakfast	Snack	Lunch	Snack	Dinner	Snack

Water Intake:

Exercise:

Day 26 – You Are Who You Are For a Reason

No, don't say that. Who are you, a mere human being, to argue with God? Should the thing that was created say to the one who created it, "Why have you made me like this?" Romans 9:20 NLT

Do you ever wonder why God made you the way He did? Why you have the body, the skin tone, the hair you have; or why you were born into the family you were born into? It was no mistake. God didn't get distracted and place you in the wrong family or wrong body. You are who you are for a reason.

I am the youngest of five children and weight wise, even as a child, the largest of all five. I am 6 years younger than my youngest middle sibling and 16 years younger than my oldest sibling. So with the age difference, you would think looking at pictures of us, I would be the smallest person in the picture. I was looking at a picture of my next to the oldest sister, my only brother, and me; I think they were in high school and I was in elementary school, but, I was wider than them!

My three oldest siblings passed away when I was in high school, and both of my parents passed away when I was 32 years old (we'll talk about this another day). I'm not able to compare myself physically to them any longer. It's just my sister Tina and I that remains of the Jones clan. But, none of them were obese like me.

So, why am I obese? This is a question I've asked myself. I don't have an answer. But, what I do know is that God says I am fearfully and wonderfully made; that I am the apple of His eye; that I am His beloved daughter and that no matter what He loves me with everlasting, unconditional love, regardless of what I look like.

Take comfort in knowing you are who you are for a reason. God placed you right where you are in that family, in that body, at this time, for a reason. You are not a mistake.

Prayer: God, thank you for giving me this body, my family and for loving me unconditionally.

Journal Your Journey: Have you ever wondered why God made you the way He did? Why you have the body, the skin tone, the hair you have; or why you were born into the family you were born into?

ME < GOD

Journal Your Journey:

Track Your Day - Date: _____/_____/_____

Breakfast	Snack	Lunch	Snack	Dinner	Snack

Water Intake:
🥛 🥛 🥛 🥛 🥛 🥛 🥛

Exercise:

Day 27 – Nothing Can Separate You From His Love

For I am convinced that neither death nor life, neither angels nor demons, neither the present nor the future, nor any powers, neither height nor depth, nor anything else in all creation, will be able to separate us from the love of God that is in Christ Jesus our Lord. Romans 8:38-39 NIV

In this day and age when the images we see on TV and in social media can cause us to question and compare ourselves to others and to strive for something that isn't real; know that God is real and never changing.

This covers every aspect of our lives. The things we've done or not done in the past; currently doing or not doing; or will or won't do in the future. Those things we've thought or done and never uttered a word about to anyone. Those things that we've done and everyone knows about. They can't and won't separate us from the love of God.

I don't know about you, but there is so much peace and comfort in knowing that no matter what, nothing can separate me from the love of God.

Prayer: Thank you, God, that nothing, absolutely nothing or anyone will ever separate me from your love.

Journal Your Journey: Do you believe that nothing will separate you from the love of God?

ME < GOD

Journal Your Journey:

Track Your Day - Date: _____/_____/_____

Breakfast	Snack	Lunch	Snack	Dinner	Snack

Water Intake:
☐ ☐ ☐ ☐ ☐ ☐ ☐

Exercise:

Day 28 - Vantage Point

"My thoughts are nothing like your thoughts," says the Lord. "And my ways are far beyond anything you could imagine. For just as the heavens are higher than the earth, so my ways are higher than your ways and my thoughts higher than your thoughts. Isaiah 55:8-9 NLT

A recent message at church was called Vantage Point. The pastor talked about how God's viewpoint of our lives is so much greater than ours. He doesn't see things from our perspective. He has the vantage point, which is a place or position where there is a broader view.

When it comes to being successful at losing weight, find the support that you can call on that has the vantage point regarding your journey. Someone who has been successful at losing weight and keeping it off. Their experience can be valuable and their encouragement priceless.

Being willing to rely on others requires humility, vulnerability, and honesty. This can be difficult if it isn't something you are used to or if you are used to going it alone. Remember that someone with a vantage point will see things from a broader perspective.

Prayer: God, thank you for reminding me that your thoughts are greater than mine and that you have a broader view than I do. Thank you for bringing the right supportive people in my life – people who have…a vantage point.

Journal Your Journey: Are you being vulnerable and honest about your weight loss journey with someone?

ME < GOD

Journal Your Journey:

Track Your Day - Date: _____/_____/_____

Breakfast	Snack	Lunch	Snack	Dinner	Snack

Water Intake:
◯ ◯ ◯ ◯ ◯ ◯ ◯

Exercise:

Day 29 – Let God Transform You

Don't copy the behavior and customs of this world, but let God transform you into a new person by changing the way you think. Then you will learn to know God's will for you, which is good and pleasing and perfect. Romans 12:2 NLT

According to data from the National Health and Nutrition Examination Survey, more than 2 in 3 (66%) adults were considered to be overweight or have obesity. According to data by Marketdata Enterprises, a market research firm that specializes in tracking niche industries, Americans spend north of $60 billion annually on everything from paying for gym memberships and joining weight-loss programs to drinking diet soda, to try to lose weight.

It makes me sad and angry at the same time to hear these statistics or facts. Sad, because I know what it feels like to be overweight and obese and how desperately you desire to change and how hard it can be to change, and knowing that so many other people are struggling with these same feelings. Angry, because the weight loss industry is big business capitalizing off of the pain of others and for many of these businesses it is a false promise of quick and rapid weight loss which doesn't last.

I fell into the trap of copying the behavior and customs of this world; large portions, modern conveniences that minimize (darn near eliminates) the need for movement; and instant self-gratification. These behaviors and customs contributed significantly to my being overweight and obese. But, I have yielded to God, and I am allowing Him to change me, transform me, and change my thinking. I am learning to know His will for me, and my hope is that you will too, my friend.

Prayer: God, I no longer copy the behaviors and customs of this world. Thank you for revealing your pleasing and perfect will for me.

Journal Your Journey: Have you copied the behaviors and customs of this world?

ME < GOD

Journal Your Journey:

Track Your Day - Date: _____/_____/_____

Breakfast	Snack	Lunch	Snack	Dinner	Snack

Water Intake:
◯ ◯ ◯ ◯ ◯ ◯ ◯

Exercise:

Day 30 – Let's Celebrate Together!

"The master was full of praise. 'Well done, my good and faithful servant. You have been faithful in handling this small amount, so now I will give you many more responsibilities. Let's celebrate together!' Matthew 25:21 NLT

We are 30 days into this journey of less of you and more of God. That calls for a celebration! No matter where you are on this journey, just starting out or at your goal or destination, you should celebrate what you have accomplished.

A friend of mine created a non-profit organization called Celebrate Me. She started this organization to help recognize and celebrate people's accomplishments. She believed that many people were like her and didn't celebrate themselves when they achieved a goal but instead downplayed it and kept pressing towards the next thing.

God believes in celebrations. There are many celebrations throughout the Bible. In the parable of the three servants whose master entrusted them with his property the master celebrated with the two servants who were diligent with what they were given; although their results differed, he celebrated the accomplishments of both. So, don't feel guilty about celebrating your accomplishments. Do something to reward yourself and share it with others.

Prayer: God, thank you for reminding me to celebrate my accomplishments.

Journal Your Journey: How are you going to celebrate your accomplishments?

ME < GOD

Journal Your Journey:

Track Your Day - Date: _____/_____/_____

Breakfast	Snack	Lunch	Snack	Dinner	Snack

Water Intake: ◯ ◯ ◯ ◯ ◯ ◯ ◯

Exercise:

ME < GOD

Voyage
Two

(voy•age — an account of a journey)

Day 31 – What You Need To Know When You Need To Know It

Now we see things imperfectly, like puzzling reflections in a mirror, but then we will see everything with perfect clarity. All that I know now is partial and incomplete, but then I will know everything completely, just as God now knows me completely. 1 Corinthians 13:12 NLT

The way we see ourselves usually isn't the way others see us. I am often surprised by the things people say to me about how I've impacted their lives and especially those I've only known for a short period of time. I always attribute that to the spirit of God living in me.

As your body is changing and there is less of you physically, and spiritually more of God, you will learn more and more about Him, His word, and His ways. I love those moments when I go, "Oh, so that's why you had me in that place at that time God!"

There will come a time when you will know everything completely, just as God knows you completely. He loves you so much, and He knows when it is best for you to have the whole picture. In the meantime, trust Him and allow Him to lead you.

Prayer: Thank you, God, for revealing to me what I need to know when I need to know it and for guiding me through this journey.

Journal Your Journey: Do you trust God that he will reveal to you what you need to know, when you need to know it?

ME < GOD

Journal Your Journey:

Track Your Day - Date: _____/_____/_____

Breakfast	Snack	Lunch	Snack	Dinner	Snack

Water Intake:

Exercise:

Day 32 – Ask, Using His Name

You haven't done this before. Ask, using my name, and you will receive, and you will have abundant joy. John 16:24 NLT

I've spent the majority of my life struggling with losing weight. When I became a believer in 2001 and started learning about God and building our relationship, I was so excited, and I knew my life would never be the same. What I didn't know and have learned over time is that God cares about everything I care about, because He cares for me. It wasn't until recently that I realized this includes my struggle with my weight.

Jesus was explaining to the disciples in John 16 that soon He'd be going away and what was going to happen with their relationship with Him and the Father. The dynamic was about to change, they'd have direct access to the Father by asking and using His name, Jesus.

The dynamic has changed when it comes to the struggle with my weight. I've always had access to our Father since accepting Jesus as my Lord and Savior, but I had kept this part of me to myself and not asked in Jesus' name for help to lose the weight. Perhaps you haven't done this before either. His word says we can ask using His name, and we will not only receive, but we'll have abundant joy!

Prayer: God, thank you for caring for me and giving me the ability to ask for help with my weight loss. In Jesus' name. Amen.

Journal Your Journey: Have you asked in Jesus' name for help to lose weight?

ME < GOD

Journal Your Journey:

Track Your Day - Date: _____/_____/_____

Breakfast	Snack	Lunch	Snack	Dinner	Snack

Water Intake:

Exercise:

Day 33 – Not What You Did or How You Look

God saved you by his grace when you believed. And you can't take credit for this; it is a gift from God. Salvation is not a reward for the good things we have done, so none of us can boast about it. For we are God's masterpiece. He has created us anew in Christ Jesus, so we can do the good things he planned for us long ago. Ephesians 2:8-10 NLT

It can be hard to just accept the love of Christ because we live in a world where what we do or don't do impacts how we are loved by others, paid, rewarded or not at work and how we live. So, it can be a foreign concept to accept that, nothing we have done or can do will change God's love for us.

We even routinely judge ourselves based on how we look or feel. When we look at ourselves in the mirror, and we like what we see, we feel more worthy of love from God or others. Conversely, when we don't like what we see, we may feel less worthy of love.

God wants us to redirect what we look at; instead of looking at ourselves to judge whether we are worthy, look at Him and believe He made us worthy. He has clothed us in His righteousness and in His perfect love. It wasn't based on anything we did or how we look, it is freely given to us by His grace when we believe.

Prayer: Thank you, God, that by your grace I am saved and loved, and nothing will change that because I believe.

Journal Your Journey: Have you been judging yourself based on how you look?

ME < GOD

Journal Your Journey:

Track Your Day - Date: _____/_____/_____

Breakfast	Snack	Lunch	Snack	Dinner	Snack

Water Intake:

Exercise:

Day 34 – Every Detail of Your Life

The Lord directs the steps of the godly. He delights in every detail of their lives. Though they stumble, they will never fall, for the Lord holds them by the hand. Psalm 37:23-24 NLT

It can be easy to get bored with eating the same, or similar things that you know will help you lose weight, so you desire to switch it up or add some variety. There are many ways to add variety and still stay on your plan, and usually, there are others who have felt the same way and posted suggestions on a social media site on how they mixed it up.

God knows there are times where you are going to be focused and flowing along with no problems on this journey, and although He could make it like that all the time, He knows that you grow more when you rely on Him during those times that it isn't so easy or when it is arduous.

I routinely take verses out of the Bible and personalize them to me, so that I remember that God is speaking directly to me. Today's verse always makes me happy because I know all too well how on this journey I've stumbled or been bored, but I know that He is with me.

Prayer: Thank you, Lord, that you direct my steps and delight in every detail of my life. Though I stumble, I will never fall, for you hold me by my hand!

Journal Your Journey: Do you realize that God delights in every detail of your life?

ME < GOD

Journal Your Journey:

Track Your Day - Date: _____/_____/_____

Breakfast	Snack	Lunch	Snack	Dinner	Snack

Water Intake:

Exercise:

Day 35 – Ask Questions

"Sir," Gideon replied, "if the Lord is with us, why has all this happened to us? And where are all the miracles our ancestors told us about? Didn't they say, 'The Lord brought us up out of Egypt'? But now the Lord has abandoned us and handed us over to the Midianites." Judges 6:13 NLT

I have been wondering how I got here, as in a place where I have so much belly fat or fat in general. I guess theoretically I know it is consuming more calories than I expend on a daily basis, or eating too much and not enough exercise (no exercise for the majority of my life). But, my mind is still puzzled about why some people are naturally slim, and some aren't. How did I get into the "aren't" group, Lord?

I am working diligently to lose weight and seeing progress. But, it's like Wow… I really have to lose this much weight God? How did I get here? You may have similar thoughts or questions for God; just like Gideon in this passage of scripture, He welcomes our questions and isn't upset or impatient with us when we ask them; or He doesn't think it is a dumb question or thought.

One thing I think we all know is that we can't keep doing the same things and expecting different results. Yet, many of us have done that for years when it comes to our weight loss journey. My hope for you is that you will have a conversation with God; ask the questions you have about your journey, seek Him for the answer, and that from this experience you walk away changed.

Prayer: God, thank you for giving me a safe place to ask questions that I wouldn't ask anyone else; and for giving me insight that transforms me.

Journal Your Journey: What questions do you have for God about your weight loss journey?

ME < GOD

Journal Your Journey:

Track Your Day - Date: _____/_____/_____

Breakfast	Snack	Lunch	Snack	Dinner	Snack

Water Intake:
🥛 🥛 🥛 🥛 🥛 🥛 🥛

Exercise:

Day 36 – The Mud & The Mire

He lifted me out of the pit of despair, out of the mud and the mire. He set my feet on solid ground and steadied me as I walked along. He has given me a new song to sing, a hymn of praise to our God. Many will see what he has done and be amazed. They will put their trust in the Lord. Psalm 40:2-3 NLT

This journey can be challenging, and there are times that you will be sad and feel despair or be bogged down with self-pity over the difficulty of losing weight. Especially when you feel like you've done everything right and the scale doesn't move. But, self-pity can be a very slippery slope to a bottomless pit you don't want to be in.

Just know my friend you are not alone. I have felt this way and so have many others. God's reach is long enough to rescue you. His light shines down on us when we are in this pit, and as we focus on His presence and trust Him, He pulls us up out of despair and gives us hope again.

In addition to practicing being in God's presence, one of the ways I've climbed out of the pit of self-pity is to help someone else. Being God's hands and feet, loving on others and serving others makes it challenging to focus on feeling sorry for yourself and your circumstances. You inevitably show others how to put their trust in the Lord, through your example.

Prayer: God, thank you for your presence especially when I am feeling sad or discouraged and for using me to be a blessing to others.

Journal Your Journey: Have you been in the pit of self-pity? If so, how do you get out?

ME < GOD

Journal Your Journey:

Track Your Day - Date: _____/_____/_____

Breakfast	Snack	Lunch	Snack	Dinner	Snack

Water Intake:
🥛 🥛 🥛 🥛 🥛 🥛 🥛 🥛

Exercise:

Day 37 – A Divine Process

For God is working in you, giving you the desire and the power to do what pleases him. Philippians 2:13 NLT

Losing weight is a slow and challenging process. Given how quickly we can gain it, it seems unbalanced that it takes much longer to lose it. The process consists of taking small positive action steps on a consistent basis over a period of time, and the weight comes off. The step you take today won't show any progress today, but those daily steps combined over time result in progress.

If you don't accept the reality of how this process works, you will struggle with maintaining results. Human nature will cause us to act for a period of time, and once we see some results we stop doing the action steps that got us those results, and then we fall back into our old way of doing things. That is why seeing it as a long-term process versus short-term; a lifestyle change versus a temporary change is essential to success. Finding what works for you and being able to incorporate it into your everyday life will ensure your success.

Our relationship with Christ is a similar process in that we are saved once, but it is a journey to becoming the new creation we already are in Christ. This process happens over time through spending time with God daily, getting to know His word and His way and allowing Him to lead us as we become more like Him. It is a divine process, where you may not notice changes in yourself daily, but with consistency over time in Christ, you look up, and you behave and act differently as a result of your daily time with Him.

Prayer: God, thank you for the process, the journey, my spiritual growth, and my mindset change about my weight loss.

Journal Your Journey: Have you accepted losing weight and keeping it off requires a lifestyle change long-term?

ME < GOD

Journal Your Journey:

Track Your Day - Date: _____/_____/_____

Breakfast	Snack	Lunch	Snack	Dinner	Snack

Water Intake:

Exercise:

Day 38 – See Yourself As He Sees You

But the Lord said to Samuel, "Don't judge by his appearance or height, for I have rejected him. The Lord doesn't see things the way you see them. People judge by outward appearance, but the Lord looks at the heart." 1 Samuel 16:7 NLT

Are you your own worst critic? Do you say nicer things to others than you say to yourself? If so, my friend, you are not alone. I am a natural encourager. I can always find the positive in someone's situation, and I will encourage them. Now, when it comes to seeing the positive in my own personal circumstances, not so much.

I recently had my husband take pictures of me to chronicle my weight loss journey, and he had taken pictures of me approximately 30 days before. As I viewed both sets of pictures, I couldn't see any difference or change in my body and my husband was shocked. He pointed out the changes he saw and kept asking me, "Do you not see that?" I couldn't see it.

God doesn't see us the way we see ourselves. He sees us as we really are, made in His image.

Prayer: God, thank you for seeing me through your eyes and showing me how to see myself as you see me.

Journal Your Journey: How do you see yourself?

ME < GOD

Journal Your Journey:

Track Your Day - Date: _____/_____/_____

Breakfast	Snack	Lunch	Snack	Dinner	Snack

Water Intake: ☐ ☐ ☐ ☐ ☐ ☐ ☐

Exercise:

Day 39 – More Than Anything

"All right then," Joshua said, "destroy the idols among you, and turn your hearts to the Lord, the God of Israel." Joshua 24:23 NLT

I was listening to the song "More Than Anything" by Natalie Grant on the radio today. It says help me want the healer more than the healing; help me want the Savior more than the saving; help me want the giver more than the giving; help me want you, Jesus, more than anything.

I have desired for so long to lose weight, and although I know God can do anything, I finally want the Creator more than the weight loss; I want Jesus more than anything. If I never lose another pound, I'll be okay, but I won't be okay without Jesus. He loves me when I don't; He is faithful when I am faithless; He gives me grace when I don't deserve it. He is everything.

It's not that God doesn't want us to desire to lose weight or the many other things our hearts desire. He wants us to put it in the proper order and to not place anything above Him. Our greatest desire should be for Him. Everything else is temporary, but His love never fails. It is everlasting.

Prayer: Thank you God for helping me to want you more than anything.

Journal Your Journey: Are you desiring to lose weight more than you desire God?

ME < GOD

Journal Your Journey:

Track Your Day - Date: _____/_____/_____

Breakfast	Snack	Lunch	Snack	Dinner	Snack

Water Intake:
☐ ☐ ☐ ☐ ☐ ☐

Exercise:

Day 40 – It is Possible

He replied, "What is impossible for people is possible with God." Luke 18:27 NLT

I went to lunch recently with two colleagues I met in a company training. We went to a Mexican restaurant, and they ordered and ate some of the things I would usually eat; but because I am on my specific eating plan, I didn't. I remained disciplined.

I shared with them about my weight loss journey, and they commended me for being diligent and disciplined. When we got back to class, one of the ladies shared with me that she had lost over 100 pounds. Of course, I was excited for her. I was intrigued and wanted to hear about her journey. She said with some trepidation, "I had gastric bypass surgery. I don't necessarily regret it, but I wish I had lost it the way you're doing it."

Society and modern conveniences have caused us to seek instant gratification in so many areas of our lives. It can cause us to think or feel like there are no options or other ways of doing things or to have a sense that time is not on our side. This is a deceptive practice that the enemy uses.

With God all things are possible. We don't have to believe the lies the enemy tries to tell us; such as you'll never lose the weight. Even if you have accepted the lies and acted upon them; know that there is no condemnation to those who are in Christ Jesus. Refocus on the truth, what God says and keep moving forward. You can lose the weight; it is possible with God.

Prayer: God, thank you for making my permanent weight loss possible. No matter how many times I've tried and gained it back, I know with you all things are possible.

Journal Your Journey: Do you believe it is possible to lose the weight you want to lose and keep it off?

ME < GOD

Journal Your Journey:

___

Track Your Day - Date: _____/_____/_____

Breakfast	Snack	Lunch	Snack	Dinner	Snack

Water Intake:
☐ ☐ ☐ ☐ ☐ ☐ ☐

Exercise:

Day 41 – In Spite of Temptation

Keep watch and pray, so that you will not give in to temptation. For the spirit is willing, but the body is weak!" Matthew 26:41 NLT

Recently we had house guests, my sister-in-law, and niece. I was excited that they were coming to stay with us because we enjoy spending time with our family. It is especially lovely when they are mindful of what they eat too! My sister-in-law recently lost 50 pounds, and she has changed her lifestyle to eat healthier.

A confession I've made is, 'When I sit down to eat at no time do I allow anyone else to influence, tempt, or discourage me in any negative way.' It has not always been that way. In the past, I've allowed my husband, family, and friends to influence what I ate negatively and vice versus, I'm sure. Especially at family gatherings or parties where there is usually unhealthy food and desserts. I've grown, and I now have conviction and confidence regarding what I will and won't eat, and no one can influence it, except God.

Perhaps you have always had this conviction, or you are just starting to get to that place on your journey where you don't allow anyone to influence, tempt, or discourage you in any negative way. Either way, this conviction is key to weight loss success.

Prayer: Lord, thank you for giving me the conviction to stick with my eating plan in spite of the temptations that come my way.

Journal Your Journey: Do you have conviction to stick to your eating plan in spite of temptation?

ME < GOD

Journal Your Journey:

Track Your Day - Date: _____/_____/_____

Breakfast	Snack	Lunch	Snack	Dinner	Snack

Water Intake:
◯ ◯ ◯ ◯ ◯ ◯ ◯

Exercise:

Day 42 – Freedom to Choose

"You are a witness to your own decision," Joshua said. "You have chosen to serve the Lord." "Yes," they replied, "we are witnesses to what we have said." Joshua 24:22 NLT

We were at a mall in Birmingham spending time with family, and we thought it would be a great choice to eat at the food court so that everyone could find what they wanted to eat. I stopped eating meat almost a year and a half ago, and it is difficult to find ample options to eat when I am out.

The decision to not eat meat isn't a popular one, and it has been somewhat of a fad for some since watching the documentary "What the Health," which promotes a plant-based diet. But, I've never been much of a meat eater, so it came naturally to me to make the transition. It is a matter of preference, and I prefer and choose not to eat meat.

Life is full of choices, and we make them every day. God allows us to choose. He urges us to choose life with Him. We can make this choice by loving the Lord our God, obeying Him, and committing ourselves firmly to Him. This is the best choice I have ever made in my life. My hope my friend, is that if you haven't already chosen, that you make the same decision. I am confident that your life will never be the same and you won't ever regret it. If you have already chosen life with Him, continue to make that choice every day.

Prayer: God, thank you for giving us the freedom to choose and showing us how to continue to chose life with you every day.

Journal Your Journey: Have you chosen life with God?

ME < GOD

Journal Your Journey:

Track Your Day - Date: _____/_____/_____

Breakfast	Snack	Lunch	Snack	Dinner	Snack

Water Intake:
⌴ ⌴ ⌴ ⌴ ⌴ ⌴

Exercise:

Day 43 – Benefits in This Life & The Life to Come

"Physical training is good, but training for godliness is much better, promising benefits in this life and in the life to come." 1 Timothy 4:8 NLT

I have been exercising consistently at least four to seven times a week for over a year. I enjoy exercise. But, I prefer to do it in the comfort of my own home. I don't like the idea of getting up, getting dressed and driving to the gym. It has worked well for me to use DVDs and videos on YouTube to workout. I never have an excuse, not to workout; whether it is raining, snowing or I'm out of town, and I can exercise.

Though they work in conjunction, and working out is an integral part of my overall health; I've learned that eating right is far more critical. This is similar to our spiritual life. Physically training our bodies is good for our overall health, but spiritual training in Godliness is much better. Because as we physically train our bodies, it is good for right now and for the future, but it is temporary; it is for our time in this world. Spiritual training is for right now, the future, and for eternity.

Spiritual training can take place anywhere you are, as long as you are in the presence of God. At church, at home, in the car, in another country, anywhere. So, do both my friend, physically and spiritually train, wherever is most comfortable for you, but know that your spiritual training will last forever.

Prayer: God, thank you for giving me the desire to physically and spiritually train, knowing that training for Godliness is much better, promising benefits in this life and in the life to come.

Journal Your Journey: Have you committed to spiritually and physically training yourself?

ME < GOD

Journal Your Journey:

Track Your Day - Date: _____/_____/_____

Breakfast	Snack	Lunch	Snack	Dinner	Snack

Water Intake:
⌂ ⌂ ⌂ ⌂ ⌂ ⌂ ⌂

Exercise:

Day 44 – Wonderfully Complex

You made all the delicate, inner parts of my body and knit me together in my mother's womb. Thank you for making me so wonderfully complex! Your workmanship is marvelous—how well I know it. Psalm 139:13-14 NLT

I recently watched a reality game show, and there was an intense discussion between two of the participants about derogatory names people have called them. They were having an honest and challenging conversation riddled with the pain of their personal experiences. It made me sad thinking about the pain many of us have suffered at the carelessness and unfortunately intentional words people say, myself included.

Being overweight and being dark skinned, are two things that have brought about name-calling throughout my life. When society places a higher value on being thin and light or white, you have to be secure in who God made you to be. The images we see in magazines, on television, or in other forms of media, don't commonly show overweight, or people of color, in a favorable way as often as the images of thin, light-skinned, or white people.

When people call us names and those names cause us to feel insecure because we start believing the lies that we've heard; we have to remember the truth and tell ourselves the truth. God sees us all as we really are, His beloved children; made in His image, beautiful, perfect, and wonderfully made.

Prayer: God, thank you for telling me the truth about me; and helping me to always believe your word concerning me, regardless of the names others call me.

Journal Your Journey: Do you believe what God says about you more than what others say about you?

ME < GOD

Journal Your Journey:

Track Your Day - Date: _____/_____/_____

Breakfast	Snack	Lunch	Snack	Dinner	Snack

Water Intake:

Exercise:

Day 45 - Day & Night

Study this Book of Instruction continually. Meditate on it day and night so you will be sure to obey everything written in it. Only then will you prosper and succeed in all you do. Joshua 1:8 NLT

There is a concept called the lead-lag effect. There are lead activities you do that are correlated with lag results. In this weight loss journey, some lead activities are eating nutritious food or exercising daily. If you do these lead activities, the lag results will manifest, such as weighing less or being fit and toned. When the lead activities are not taking place, you cannot expect to see any of the lag results.

The lead-lag effect applies in many areas of our lives, including our relationship with God. Some examples of lead activities are meditating, reading and studying His word, spending time in His presence, and prayer; which manifest lag results: increased faith, wisdom, and the fruit of the Spirit. However, there are times in the Kingdom of God that there is no need for any lead activities and there are just results; those are miracles! Because at any time our God is able to do more than we can ask or think.

God tells us a couple of times in the Bible to meditate in His word continually, day and night (lead activities), and that it will bring us great success (lag results). Lead activities produce good habits. The discipline that is practiced by doing lead activities builds a desire to be engaged in healthy habits daily. Lag results are a natural by product. If you are struggling to find the time or be consistent with your lead activities, whether on your spiritual or weight loss journey, talk with God about your schedule and how to reprioritize. It will be the best planning meeting you've ever had.

Prayer: God, help me to reprioritize my daily life to make time for the lead activities that will bring me success in all areas of my life.

Journal Your Journey: Have you identified the lead activities you should do regularly to get the lag results you want?

ME < GOD

Journal Your Journey:

Track Your Day - Date: _____/_____/_____

Breakfast	Snack	Lunch	Snack	Dinner	Snack

Water Intake:
⌂ ⌂ ⌂ ⌂ ⌂ ⌂ ⌂

Exercise:

Day 46 – Diligent & Prepared

Five of them were foolish, and five were wise. The five who were foolish didn't take enough olive oil for their lamps, but the other five were wise enough to take along extra oil. Matthew 25:2-4 NLT

It can be mundane to do the same things over and over again. Some days I am excited about my daily routine, then there are other days where I am like really this again today! But my daily routine has helped me to be diligent and ready at all times. I had an all-day team meeting at my company's corporate office in Raleigh, so I had to travel from my town, north of Atlanta to Raleigh. It could have been easy for me to not maintain my daily routine because I was traveling. But, I brought my meal replacements with me, and I went to the store once I got checked in to my hotel, to get other liquid items I needed that I couldn't bring on the plane.

It is a blessing to have your meals provided and paid for by your company. It is only a concern if you don't eat what is offered. Breakfast was an assortment of large muffins, and lunch was a box lunch with deli sandwiches. I am Pescatarian, a person who does not eat meat but eats fish, so there was nothing provided that I'd eat. I was able to maintain my routine because I had prepared and brought what I needed with me.

How are you doing with your daily routine? Are you prepared at all times to have what you need for your weight loss success? God tells us through parables to be prepared for His return. One of my favorite parables is that of the wise and foolish virgins or bridesmaids. In the parable the bridegroom's arrival was sure; just like your need to eat a meal is certain, and Christ's return is certain. What wasn't certain was when the bridegroom would come, or when Christ will return, or when someone else is providing your meals, whether it will be what you need. Thus, unlike the five foolish virgins, we have to be consistently diligent.

Prayer: God, help me to be wise, diligent and prepared for my daily routine and your return.

Journal Your Journey: How are you doing with your daily routine? Are you prepared at all times to have what you need for weight loss success?

ME < GOD

Journal Your Journey:

Track Your Day - Date: _____ / _____ / _____

Breakfast	Snack	Lunch	Snack	Dinner	Snack

Water Intake:

Exercise:

Day 47 – Made in His Image

So God created human beings in his own image. In the image of God he created them; male and female he created them. Genesis 1:27 NLT

I recently watched the movie, "I Feel Pretty." It was about a woman who struggled with feeling insecure and inadequate. She fell and hit her head, and after her fall, even though she was looking at herself in the mirror, her head injury caused her to see herself as beautiful, capable, and full of confidence. This change in her perspective caused her life to completely change and for other people to see her differently as well.

This movie reminded me of several key things. First, how we see ourselves and if we exude confidence, has a lot to do with how others see us. As well as, Eleanor Roosevelt's quote- No one can make you feel inferior without your consent. Lastly, it doesn't matter what you look like, you can be confident in who God made you to be; He doesn't make mistakes. God is waiting for us to be, and live, as He created us. That means believing the truth of His word and not the lies the enemy or the world has told us.

Prayer: God, thank you for making me in your image, and that I can be confident in who I am.

Journal Your Journey: Are you confident in who God made you to be regardless of how you look?

ME < GOD

Journal Your Journey:

Track Your Day - Date: _____/_____/_____

Breakfast	Snack	Lunch	Snack	Dinner	Snack

Water Intake: ⛁ ⛁ ⛁ ⛁ ⛁ ⛁ ⛁

Exercise:

Day 48 – He Knows Everything About You

O Lord, you have examined my heart and know everything about me. You know when I sit down or stand up. You know my thoughts even when I'm far away. You see me when I travel and when I rest at home. You know everything I do. You know what I am going to say even before I say it, Lord. You go before me and follow me. You place your hand of blessing on my head. Such knowledge is too wonderful for me, too great for me to understand! Psalm 139:1-6 NLT

I have always found it interesting how many of us try to fix ourselves or clean ourselves up before coming to God, when He is the one that does the fixing and cleaning up way better than we could. Equally interesting to me is how many of us separate parts of our lives from God as though He doesn't already know or care about it.

God knows everything about us, more than we know about ourselves, and He loves us deeply and unconditionally despite anything we think would cause Him to not love us. You can talk to Him, bring to Him, and share with Him, absolutely anything and everything!

When we try to hide hurt or pain we feel about something that happened to us, it just festers and impacts other areas of our lives. A sin we commit that we think no one knows about can control us or cause us to live a double life, and we may not even realize it. Believe me, my friend, God already knows, and He still loves you.

Prayer: God, thank you for reminding me that I don't have to hide anything from you because you already know it.

Journal Your Journey: Are you trying to hide how you feel or what you have done from God?

ME < GOD

Journal Your Journey:

Track Your Day - Date: _____/_____/_____

Breakfast	Snack	Lunch	Snack	Dinner	Snack

Water Intake:

Exercise:

Day 49 – In His Presence

You will show me the way of life, granting me the joy of your presence and the pleasures of living with you forever. Psalm 16:11 NLT

I was on a monthly video call that I have with a group of amazing women, and our guest speaker was sharing with us about being in the secret place with God and how this prepares us to do His will and be at peace no matter what is going on around us or happening to us.

One of the ladies asked a great question, "What do you do when life's challenges or your crazy schedule keeps you from spending time with God in the secret place consistently?" Another one of the ladies answered and said, "We all go through seasons in our lives where time is limited, so remember that God is always with us. We can experience His presence any time."

Whether you've had a baby, started a new relationship and trying to figure out how to balance time between work, family and existing friends, or started a new weight loss program and trying to fit in exercise. Whatever is causing you to not find the time, remember that God is always with you and you can be in His presence when nursing your baby, spending time with a new friend, or exercising; He is always there.

Also, if you ever feel condemned for not spending more time with God, know that His word says there is no condemnation to those who are in Christ Jesus.

So my friend, make it a habit to spend time with God in the secret place, and when there isn't time available, remember to practice being in His presence in the midst of what you are doing, even exercise!

Prayer: God, thank you for the joy I find in your presence and that I can be in your presence whenever and wherever.

Journal Your Journey: Are you practicing being in God's presence wherever you are or during whatever it is you are doing?

ME < GOD

Journal Your Journey:

Track Your Day - Date: _____/_____/_____

Breakfast	Snack	Lunch	Snack	Dinner	Snack

Water Intake: ☐ ☐ ☐ ☐ ☐ ☐ ☐

Exercise:

Day 50 – Changing Your Thoughts & Actions

Since you have heard about Jesus and have learned the truth that comes from him, throw off your old sinful nature and your former way of life, which is corrupted by lust and deception. Instead, let the Spirit renew your thoughts and attitudes. Put on your new nature, created to be like God—truly righteous and holy. Ephesians 4:21-24 NLT

Losing weight requires a mindset change. Keeping it off requires a lifestyle change. Therefore, long-term success requires both. Experts on WebMD say that 80% of people who successfully lose at least 10% of their body weight will gradually regain it to end up as large or even larger than they were before they went on a diet. I'm no expert, but this has been my experience. I've lost and gained weight many times.

I was talking with a few ladies one day that I had not seen in several months. They noticed how much weight I had lost and asked me how I did it. I shared my journey over the past year and the two programs I had used. One of the ladies shared with us that she was taking a shot that was helping her with her weight loss. She had lost twenty pounds in two weeks. A couple of the other ladies told her she was losing weight too fast.

I know what it's like to have such a desire to lose weight and wanting a magic pill or quick fix that will take the weight off. But, the reality is that losing weight quickly through diet pills or a fad diet plan usually won't result in long-term weight loss success. You have to decide if you want short-term or long-term results. Long-term results come through making a conscious effort to change your lifestyle, change your thoughts, and change your daily actions. It is the same when building a relationship with God. Long-term success comes from allowing God to change your heart, which comes through daily actions such as spending time in His word, in prayer, and allowing His Holy Spirit to lead you.

Prayer: God, thank you for changing my thoughts and actions to line up with my desire to lose weight and keep it off and for changing me to be more like you.

Journal Your Journey: Do your daily actions line up with your desire to lose weight?

ME < GOD

Journal Your Journey:

Track Your Day - Date: _____/_____/_____

Breakfast	Snack	Lunch	Snack	Dinner	Snack

Water Intake: ◯ ◯ ◯ ◯ ◯ ◯ ◯

Exercise:

Day 51 – Don't Fall Into The Envy Trap

When Rachel saw that she conceived no children for Jacob, she envied her sister, and said to Jacob, "Give me children, or else I will die."Genesis 30:1 AMP

Watching other people lose weight can be motivating. But, naturally, it feels even better when you are losing weight too. There are times that we all deal with feelings of jealousy or envy; which are two different things. Jealousy is a fear of losing what you have to someone else. Envy is wanting what another person has.

It is easy to fall into the envy trap of wanting to lose weight as fast or as much as someone else. We have to remember that all of our bodies are different, and what works a certain way for one person's body may or may not work for you.

The story of Rachel and Leah demonstrate the effects of envy. Rachel was beautiful and Jacob, their husband, loved her more than Leah. So, Leah envied how much Jacob loved Rachel. Leah could have children, and Rachel envied her ability to give Jacob sons. Their desires caused both of them to act out and behave in ways I am sure they both regretted.

Just like Rachel and Leah, we have to realize that our deep desires or feelings of envy over other people's weight loss are ultimately a lack of trust in God and have nothing to do with other people. When we don't believe or trust that God loves us, knows our desires, knows what we need and when we need it, we will always be trying to do things in our own strength.

Prayer: God, help me to trust and believe that you care for me and you will bless me with my deep Godly desires in your perfect time; and if my desires don't manifest, I will trust, believe and love you anyway because I know you know what is best for me.

Journal Your Journey: Have you been envious of someone else's weight loss or how they look?

ME < GOD

Journal Your Journey:

Track Your Day - Date: _____/_____/_____

Breakfast	Snack	Lunch	Snack	Dinner	Snack

Water Intake:

Exercise:

Day 52 – Heart, Mind, & Actions in Alignment

For as he thinks in his heart, so is he [in behavior—one who manipulates]. He says to you, "Eat and drink," Yet his heart is not with you [but it is begrudging the cost]. Proverbs 23:7 AMP

There is a poem, "The Man Who Thinks He Can," by Walter D. Wintle, that is about what you think you can or can't do, and that it is a matter of your state of mind. Just as the word of God says, you can say and do one thing, but if there is something else going on in your heart that is what will dominate and control your mind and ultimately your actions.

The last stanza of the poem "The Man Who Thinks He Can" is:

Life battles don't always go
To the stronger or faster man;
But sooner or later the man who wins
Is the one who thinks he can!

Are your heart and mind set on losing weight or are you just giving it lip service? You can tell if losing weight is in your heart or mind by taking note of your daily habits or actions. Do most of them align with what you say you want?

Prayer: God, thank you for aligning my actions, and my heart and mind to match my desire to lose weight.

Journal Your Journey: Are your heart and mind set on losing weight or are you just giving it lip service?

ME < GOD

Journal Your Journey:

Track Your Day - Date: _____/_____/_____

Breakfast	Snack	Lunch	Snack	Dinner	Snack

Water Intake: ⬭ ⬭ ⬭ ⬭ ⬭ ⬭ ⬭

Exercise:

Day 53 – Disappointed, Discouraged, But Not Abandoned

We are pressed on every side by troubles, but we are not crushed. We are perplexed, but not driven to despair. We are hunted down but never abandoned by God. We get knocked down, but we are not destroyed. 2 Corinthians 4:8-9 NLT

Discouragement can be a deep wound that paralyzes you from moving forward or limiting what you think you can do. Discouragement and disappointment are common emotions, and there are a number of reasons we experience these emotions. A writer with the Association for Biblical Counselors wrote: "5 Ways to Stop Discouragement From Getting the Best of You." In the blog post, she listed 4 things that cause discouragement. Being let down by your family or friends; life circumstances, when things don't go the way you had hoped; feeling that God is against you or has forgotten about you, and being disappointed in yourself when you don't meet your own or someone else's expectations of you.

The 5 ways to stop discouragement were to first be honest with yourself about how you are feeling. Take care of your body through rest and refreshing yourself. Paying attention to your thoughts and taking them captive if they don't line up with the truth of God's word. Training yourself to see out of the two lenses of life, the temporal lens and the eternal lens. Lastly, drawing close to God, because without Him life can be unbearable.

Have you been disappointed or discouraged on your weight loss journey? I have, and of the 5 ways to stop discouragement, 2 resonate with me and have helped me to keep moving forward. Being honest with myself about how I am feeling, and drawing closer to God, because even in the midst of life's most challenging circumstances He gives me peace and joy. Find what works for you to overcome discouragement.

Prayer: God, thank you for helping me to see that it is normal to be disappointed or discouraged and that I can overcome these emotions and move forward.

Journal Your Journey: Have you been disappointed or discouraged on your weight loss journey?

ME < GOD

Journal Your Journey:

Track Your Day - Date: _____/_____/_____

Breakfast	Snack	Lunch	Snack	Dinner	Snack

Water Intake:

Exercise:

Day 54 – Nothings Too Hard

I am the Lord, the God of all living things! Is anything too hard for me? Jeremiah 32:27 CEB

A dear friend of mine recently lost her father. Shortly before that, her sister passed away. I know what that pain feels like, as I too have lived through the passing of my three oldest siblings and both my parents.

I think for years I was numb after the passing of my only brother and my two oldest sisters. All three occurred during my high school years. First my brother died in a helicopter crash off the coast of Norway when I was in 9th grade; six months later when I was in 10th grade my next to the oldest sister died in a car accident in Germany; and a year later when I was in 11th grade my oldest sister passed away due to complications with Lupus.

I have never been thin, as I mentioned earlier on, but after the loss of my siblings, I constantly struggled with my weight. Then in 2004 both of my parents passed away. My dad in April and my mom in November, both unexpectedly. I had a much better support system when my parents passed, but I was already on the weight loss roller coaster and had created such bad habits that I didn't know how to overcome them. Food gave me comfort.

It wasn't until last year, 2017 that I said no more. I will not keep going around this same old mountain. I am not a victim. I am blessed and thankful to be alive. God has sustained my sister and I. We are the only two left of my core family for a reason. I am going to do what He has called me to do and be the conqueror He created me to be.

What things in your life have caused you to hold on to your weight? We can't change what has happened to us, or what will happen in the future, but we can change how we respond or deal with it. The love of God is greater than any pain or heartache. There is nothing too hard for God, which means He can help us to overcome all of life's difficulties.

Prayer: God, thank you for being with me through all of life's difficult times and for helping me to overcome anything.

Journal Your Journey: What things have happened in your life that may have caused you to gain weight and not lose it?

ME < GOD

Journal Your Journey:

Track Your Day - Date: _____/_____/_____

Breakfast	Snack	Lunch	Snack	Dinner	Snack

Water Intake:
◯ ◯ ◯ ◯ ◯ ◯ ◯

Exercise:

Day 55 – Your Future

For I know the plans I have for you," says the Lord. "They are plans for good and not for disaster, to give you a future and a hope. Jeremiah 29:11 NLT

My sister recently celebrated her birthday. As I previously mentioned, she and I are the only two left out of my core family. My brother was 22 years old, my next to the oldest sister was 24 years old, and my oldest sister was 32 years old when they passed away. So, every birthday beyond 32 has been special for my sister and me, because there were many times we thought we wouldn't live to be older than our siblings. We were 14 and 20 years old when the first one passed away. But, here we are 32 plus 14 and 20 years of experience!

God created us all for a purpose, and we don't know how long we'll be on this side of eternity. God has a plan for you while you are here. Hopefully, you know what that plan is and you are walking in it. If you don't know what it is, it is never too late to discover God's plan for your life.

My purpose is to serve others through examples of my personal life, teaching, encouraging, and helping other people succeed. I remove burdens, restore hope and leave people in a better position, having added value to their lives. This is a part of my daily confession and affirmation. Being overweight hasn't changed my purpose, but it has hindered me from being as bold and courageous sometimes due to my lack of confidence and self-esteem.

No matter how old you are; how much weight you have to lose; or whether you are sure about why God has you here; you are here for a reason, and other people need what God has placed in you, my friend.

Prayer: God, thank you for revealing and confirming your purpose for me.

Journal Your Journey: Do you know what your purpose is?

ME < GOD

Journal Your Journey:

Track Your Day - Date: _____/_____/_____

Breakfast	Snack	Lunch	Snack	Dinner	Snack

Water Intake:

Exercise:

Day 56 – You Are Complete

And because you belong to Christ you are complete, having everything you need. Christ is ruler over every other power and authority. Colossians 2:10 ERV

The other day my husband told me he needed to tell me something. Naturally, I was bracing myself for what he had to say because it must be serious if he felt the need to announce he needed to tell me something before just telling me. He said, "I loved you before you lost weight, I love you now, and I'll still love you when you get to whatever weight you want to be at, but what I love the most about your journey is the confidence I see in you that has come back. It is so attractive."

I am so thankful for having a spouse who loves me for me, regardless of my weight. That conversation with him reminded me that losing weight is about me and no one else. But, the reality is that losing weight does impact others around you. The way you see yourself, present yourself, and treat yourself, influences how others see and treat you.

How are you treating yourself? How do you see yourself? Knowing how God sees you is the best place to start because how He sees you is the truth and you decide whether to believe it or not. You are complete in Christ, which means with Christ you have everything you need. You can be confident in that.

Prayer: God, thank you for revealing to me how you see me. I am confident in who you created me to be.

Journal Your Journey: How are you treating yourself? How do you see yourself?

ME < GOD

Journal Your Journey:

Track Your Day - Date: _____/_____/_____

Breakfast	Snack	Lunch	Snack	Dinner	Snack

Water Intake:
🥛 🥛 🥛 🥛 🥛 🥛 🥛

Exercise:

Day 57 – Choice & Decision

Today I have given you the choice between life and death, between blessings and curses. Now I call on heaven and earth to witness the choice you make. Oh, that you would choose life, so that you and your descendants might live! Deuteronomy 30:19 NLT

Even though I have lost 57 pounds, there are times I look in the mirror, and all I see is how much more weight I still have to lose. It is a goal I set for myself to lose 100 pounds, so there is no one else saying that is how much I need to lose. It is a matter of being healthy. Experts provide guidelines when it comes to what is a healthy weight, body mass index (BMI), or waist size, and I desire to reach these healthy milestones.

The process of work, diligence, discipline and time that it takes to get to a goal can be arduous. I've asked myself how it was so easy to put the weight on, but so difficult to lose it and keep it off? I think it is a matter of pleasure versus pain.

It is pleasurable to eat what you want and like, or that tastes good, but may not be good for you. It is painful to deny yourself these pleasures, to workout and to do it consistently. It all comes down to a matter of choice and making a decision.

The same is true in the Kingdom of God. It all comes down to a matter of choice and making a decision. God gives us the freedom to choose. There is great reward for making the decision to follow God and to be healthy. Which choice have you made?

Prayer: God, I chose life with you and a healthy lifestyle. Thank you for the ability to choose.

Journal Your Journey: What choice have you made?

ME < GOD

Journal Your Journey:

Track Your Day - Date: _____/_____/_____

Breakfast	Snack	Lunch	Snack	Dinner	Snack

Water Intake: ▢ ▢ ▢ ▢ ▢ ▢

Exercise:

Day 58 – A Gift From God

God saved you by his grace when you believed. And you can't take credit for this; it is a gift from God. Salvation is not a reward for the good things we have done, so none of us can boast about it. Ephesians 2:8-9 NLT

There are several people I know that are working on losing weight. Each using a different weight loss plan, and each having various levels of success. I had a discussion with one of them, and we talked about how any plan you use will probably work, as long as you work it and remain consistent. So the key is to find what works for you and stick to it. Have you found the plan that works for you?

In contrast, there is only one way to be saved. There aren't multiple plans. It isn't that any plan will work if you work it. There is just one plan. It tells us in Romans 10:9-10 that if we say with our mouths that Jesus is Lord, and believe in our heart that God raised Him from the dead, we shall be saved. I love that it is simple and that no matter who we are, what we have done or not done, we all can be saved.

Prayer: God, I believe that Jesus is Lord and that you raised Him from the dead. Thank you for saving me.

Journal Your Journey: Have you found the plan that works for you?

ME < GOD

Journal Your Journey:

Track Your Day - Date: _____/_____/_____

Breakfast	Snack	Lunch	Snack	Dinner	Snack

Water Intake:

Exercise:

Day 59 – Free of Fear

For God did not give us a spirit of timidity or cowardice or fear, but [He has given us a spirit] of power and of love and of sound judgment and personal discipline [abilities that result in a calm, well-balanced mind and self-control]. 2 Timothy 1:7 AMP

Recently, I started cleaning out my closet. Removing the larger size clothes to donate to charity and take to a consignment shop. I was hesitant at first to pack up some of the items, thinking what if I regain the weight and need these later. I had to force myself to be reminded that I will lose 100 pounds and keep it off. So, I won't be regaining this weight, and there is no need for larger sizes in my closet.

Have you been in this situation, where you fear you haven't really changed and you are going to revert back to your old habits? Have you held on to larger size clothing as a security blank out of fear of failure?

Fear involves the expectation of judgment or punishment. Once we accept Jesus as our Lord and Savior, He gives us the ability to be free of fear because He loves us and does not condemn us. So when fear creeps in, remind yourself that God didn't give you a spirit of fear and that no matter what happens He loves you, does not condemn you, and always works all things together for your good.

Prayer: God, thank you for loving me, which gives me the power to cast out fear in every situation.

Journal Your Journey: Do you fear that you haven't really changed or that you will revert back to your old habits?

ME < GOD

Journal Your Journey:

Track Your Day - Date: _____/_____/_____

Breakfast	Snack	Lunch	Snack	Dinner	Snack

Water Intake:

Exercise:

Day 60 – In All Circumstances

Be thankful in all circumstances, for this is God's will for you who belong to Christ Jesus. 1 Thessalonians 5:18 NLT

We are 60 days in! Congratulations! How are you doing? Have you noticed a change in yourself physically and spiritually? Are you expecting to reach your goal? Do you believe you'll succeed no matter what? I hope so, my friend.

God brought you to this place, at this moment in time, for a reason. He doesn't make mistakes. He knows where you are on your journey. Whether you've already reached your goal or have a ways to go, He is with you and will continue to be with you.

As you are tracking your progress, journaling your journey, and seeing less of you and more of God, thank Him for what He has done. Thanksgiving brings you in His presence; reminds you of how blessed you are, and it keeps your heart in right relationship with Him. I am so excited for you and can't wait to see what God will do in the next 30 days!

Prayer: Thank you, God! In all circumstances, I will thank you.

Journal Your Journey: What changes have you noticed in yourself physically and spiritually?

ME < GOD

Journal Your Journey:

Track Your Day - Date: _____/_____/_____

Breakfast	Snack	Lunch	Snack	Dinner	Snack

Water Intake: ▢ ▢ ▢ ▢ ▢ ▢ ▢

Exercise:

ME < GOD

Voyage Three

(voy•age — an account of a journey)

Day 61 – By Teaching, We Learn

And you should imitate me, just as I imitate Christ. 1 Corinthians 11:1 NLT

"By teaching, we learn," a Latin proverb said to have come from Seneca, a Roman philosopher. Researchers have dubbed this the "protégé effect," indicating that students who set out to teach others what they are learning, do better than students who learn just for their own sake.

Makes sense to me, and is why I have embarked on a journey to learn about optimal health, to learn myself and teach others about it. Not only will teaching others about optimal health help me to learn, but it will also help me to reach my goal of losing weight and keeping it off while helping others do the same.

I believe the ultimate form of "by teaching we learn," is being God's disciples. A disciple is a Christ follower who then teaches others how to follow Christ. Many times people learn by watching what we do more so than what we say, Which is why in ancient times being a disciple meant not just learning what the teacher or rabbi said, it meant interacting and following the practical ways of their life in hopes of becoming like them.

Who are you learning from to further develop as a Christ follower and to support your weight loss journey; but more importantly, who are you teaching knowing that it helps you to learn?

Prayer: God, thank you for my teacher(s) and bless them; and thank you for giving me the wisdom and courage to teach others.

Journal Your Journey: Who are you teaching knowing that it helps you to learn?

ME < GOD

Journal Your Journey:

Track Your Day - Date: _____/_____/_____

Breakfast	Snack	Lunch	Snack	Dinner	Snack

Water Intake:
☐ ☐ ☐ ☐ ☐ ☐ ☐

Exercise:

Day 62 – Non-Scale Victories

I have told you all this so that you may have peace in me. Here on earth you will have many trials and sorrows. But take heart, because I have overcome the world." John 16:33 NLT

Recently, my husband and I went to a basketball game at an arena in Atlanta. We've gone to other events in arenas, and in the past, I have been so uncomfortable because I barely fit in the seats. For the first time since I can remember, I was able to enjoy the game and have fun with my husband because I fit in the seat! These type of non-scale victories help make this weight loss journey so worth it.

Are you valuing and enjoying your non-scale victories? I know how exciting and frustrating at the same time looking at the scale after you weigh yourself can be. That is why you have to recognize and acknowledge the many other wins that occur along the way. Like not being out of breath once you get to the top of the stairs; taking the stairs in the first place; fitting back into a pair of pants you weren't quite sure you'd be able to wear again, or having your spouse be able to wrap their arms around you with room to spare. These are all victories and so worthy to be celebrated.

God wants us to be victorious in every area of our lives. In fact, He guarantees us victory, because He has already won on our behalf. When the enemy thought he was going to kill Jesus, but death was not the end, it was the beginning for all of us. Jesus defeated death and rose again. Because of that victory on Calvary that day, we have victory. As God's word says in this passage of scripture, take heart, you may have trials or sorrow, but know that God has overcome the world and if you are with Him, you too have this same victory.

Prayer: God, thank you for the victory! I will acknowledge and celebrate my victory.

Journal Your Journey: Are you valuing and enjoying your non-scale victories?

ME < GOD

Journal Your Journey:

Track Your Day - Date: _____/_____/_____

Breakfast	Snack	Lunch	Snack	Dinner	Snack

Water Intake:

Exercise:

Day 63 — Peaceful Harvest of Right Living

No discipline is enjoyable while it is happening—it's painful! But afterward there will be a peaceful harvest of right living for those who are trained in this way. So take a new grip with your tired hands and strengthen your weak knees. Hebrews 12:11-12 NLT

I never imagined that I'd be working out and loving it. But I have been doing some new workouts, high-intensity interval training (HITT), low impact version. I am working my way up to being able to do the regular version, which I know will take some time. These workouts have helped tremendously with reducing the inches around my waist, toning and sculpting my body.

When I started exercising, it wasn't enjoyable. Now, the more I exercise, the more I want to do it. My persistence, prayer, and confession that I exercise every day have helped to change my mind and my desire to exercise.

You may already enjoy exercise, if so great, continue to exercise and keep it in proper perspective. If you don't currently like to exercise and never find time to do it, start with short quick workouts or walks. Just like this passage of scripture says it may be painful at first, but afterward there will be a peaceful harvest of right living.

Prayer: God, thank you for a desire to be physically active every day.

Journal Your Journey: Are you being physically active on a regular basis?

ME < GOD

Journal Your Journey:

Track Your Day - Date: _____/_____/_____

Breakfast	Snack	Lunch	Snack	Dinner	Snack

Water Intake: ☐ ☐ ☐ ☐ ☐ ☐ ☐ ☐

Exercise:

Day 64 – Diligence Required

But the one who endures to the end will be saved. Matthew 24:13 NLT

I recently got into a size 14. I know for some of you that is not an accomplishment, but it is an accomplishment for me, as I haven't worn a size 14 for over 12 years. I am so excited, and I feel so blessed to be back down to a size where I can walk into any store and purchase clothes, not just a plus size store. This was one of my "whys" of why I am on this weight loss journey.

I still have a ways to go, as my waistline is larger than what is recommended to substantially reduce health risks, 31.5 inches. My primary goal is to lose 100 pounds and keep it off - 58 down, 42 more to go, but I also want to be fit and within healthy guidelines.

Revisit your "why" today. Why are you on this journey? Have you achieved some of your why so far? As you can see from my personal example, it doesn't all happen at the same time, it may be achieved in phases. Diligence is needed to reach your goals. It doesn't matter how fast you do it, just that you keep going until you accomplish your goals.

God tells us that many things will happen in the world and to us before He returns and that we are not to be distracted by these things. But, that those who endure to the end will be saved. The same is true with your weight loss journey.

Prayer: God, thank you that I will endure until the end.

Journal Your Journey: Why are you on this weight loss journey?

ME < GOD

Journal Your Journey:

Track Your Day - Date: _____/_____/_____

Breakfast	Snack	Lunch	Snack	Dinner	Snack

Water Intake:
☐ ☐ ☐ ☐ ☐ ☐ ☐

Exercise:

Day 65 – One Thing Will Never Change

Jesus Christ is the same yesterday, today, and forever. Hebrews 13:8 NLT

I am changing. Naturally, my body is physically changing as I lose weight, but my mindset is changing too. I am learning about health and nutrition, which I never knew or understood growing up. My family didn't practice, teach or model healthy habits, because they didn't know. You can't teach what you don't know.

As I am changing and desiring to be healthy and live a healthy lifestyle, I find myself in uncharted territory and asking myself what my life will look like as a healthy and fit person. What things will be different and what things will be the same?

Even though as people we grow and change, sometimes for the best and sometimes not; one thing remains the same, Jesus. He is the same yesterday, today and forever.

Prayer: Thank you, God, that you never change, and that no matter how I change, you remain the same and by my side.

Journal Your Journey: What will your life look like as a healthy and fit person? What things will be different and what things will be the same?

ME < GOD

Journal Your Journey:

Track Your Day - Date: _____/_____/_____

Breakfast	Snack	Lunch	Snack	Dinner	Snack

Water Intake:

Exercise:

Day 66 – You Have The Power

I also pray that you will understand the incredible greatness of God's power for us who believe him. This is the same mighty power that raised Christ from the dead and seated him in the place of honor at God's right hand in the heavenly realms. Ephesians 1:19-20 NLT

Some results of a lifetime of unhealthy habits are disease and sickness. I am blessed that this has not occurred in my body. I have a friend who has been diagnosed with Lupus, and she is also pre-diabetic and has been taking medication for both. I understand that she may not be able to do anything in the natural to prevent Lupus, but she has control over Type II Diabetes.

She and I were having a conversation about taking action over the things we can control. I told her that this final weight loss journey of mine was sparked by the doctor telling me my A1C level was high. The doctor said I was pre-diabetic and placed me on prescription medication. That was one of the catalysts that made me decide that anything that is within my control, I would do it to prevent this disease and losing weight was one of the most significant factors.

Alice Walker said, "The most common way people give up their power is by thinking they don't have any." You have the power to change your life. God has given you this power. As our scripture says today, I pray, my friend, that you understand the incredible greatness of God's power that is available to those of us who believe.

Prayer: God, thank you for giving me the power to change my life and to do what you've called me to do.

Journal Your Journey: Are you doing the things you have control over to lose weight and/or to prevent sickness and disease?

ME < GOD

Journal Your Journey:

Track Your Day - Date: _____ / _____ / _____

Breakfast	Snack	Lunch	Snack	Dinner	Snack

Water Intake:

Exercise:

Day 67 – Day & Night

But they delight in the law of the Lord, meditating on it day and night.
Psalm 1:2 NLT

I am in awe of God when it comes to my weight loss. I mentioned early in this book how I had settled with the fact that I was overweight and maybe for the rest of my life. I basically had lost hope, because I had tried so many times to lose weight and I would always gain it back. I know beyond a shadow of a doubt that it is different this time.

I have two Post-It notes on my bathroom mirror. One says, "I can do this" and the other says "I will do this." I put them on the mirror about four months ago. Naturally, after some time, I can walk in and not notice them at all. But, on those days when I need encouragement and to be reminded that I will lose 100 pounds and keep it off, I walk in the bathroom, and these notes are the reminder I need.

It is like that with God's word, we have to remind ourselves what it says and use the word to encourage ourselves. This is why meditation of the word is so vital to everyday victory. There are numerous times throughout the Bible where God tells us to meditate on His word, which just means to reflect on it or rehearse it over and over in our minds.

Prayer: God, thank you that as I meditate on your word, I will have great success.

Journal Your Journey: Are you using God's word to encourage yourself on your weight loss journey?

ME < GOD

Journal Your Journey:

Track Your Day - Date: _____/_____/_____

Breakfast	Snack	Lunch	Snack	Dinner	Snack

Water Intake:

Exercise:

Day 68 – You Are Redeemed

But now, this is what the Lord, your Creator says, O Jacob, And He who formed you, O Israel, "Do not fear, for I have redeemed you [from captivity]; I have called you by name; you are Mine! Isaiah 43:1 AMP

Do you ever wonder why we give more weight to what people say in society than what God says? It seems silly to me when I sit back and really think about it, because God is all powerful, all knowing, and loves us immensely. When we know this about God, I mean like it is settled in our spirit who He is; we would dare not believe what anyone else says about us that is contrary to what He says.

Are you not quite at that place my friend, where you only believe what God says about you? If so, you are not alone, because I still find myself in this place at times. This world we live in can cause us to doubt and question who and whose we are, with its images that bombard us on television, and in magazines.

That is why it is essential to be continuously connected and in tune with God to remain focused on what He says about you, so you can ingrain it in your heart and mind, which allows you to combat what you see and hear in the world. We are like Jacob, who became Israel after his night of transformation with God. God tells him to not fear, that he has been redeemed from captivity and that he is His!

We too, my friend, have been redeemed from captivity (the condition of being imprisoned or confined), whatever that means for you, whether it is your weight, the lies you've believed that other people told you or that you told yourself; be free and remember that you are His.

Prayer: God, thank you for redeeming me from being confined by my weight or anything else. I am so thankful that I am yours!

Journal Your Journey: Do you believe what God says about you?

ME < GOD

Journal Your Journey:

Track Your Day - Date: _____/_____/_____

Breakfast	Snack	Lunch	Snack	Dinner	Snack

Water Intake:
☐ ☐ ☐ ☐ ☐ ☐

Exercise:

Day 69 — Grace, Special Favor

But whatever I am now, it is all because God poured out his special favor on me—and not without results. 1 Corinthians 15:10a NLT

One of my coworkers that have been working on losing weight just celebrated a 20-pound loss. Her goal is to lose 130 pounds. She came to my office and asked: "So, when did you start to buy new clothes?" This is like one of the best feelings when you notice your body shrinking and your clothes getting too big for you!

I told her that I have purchased new clothes sporadically when I see things on sale; and that sometimes it may not be quite the size that fits comfortably yet, but I know I am headed there, and it is motivation to see it fit in a few weeks.

I have a similar feeling when I notice that God is transforming me spiritually. It is the best feeling when something that used to upset you just rolls off your back. When you used to respond in an inappropriate way when someone was negative or rude to you, and now you smile and pray for them. When things your spouse did or said made you angry or anxious, and instead of expecting him to read your mind, you calmly and clearly communicate to him how that makes you feel.

God is amazing! His love and grace change us in ways we never even knew were possible or that we even knew needed to be changed. I read a post from BibleTalkTV by Mike Mazzalonga called "The Impact of Grace." He shares how the Bible ultimately is all about the incredible story of God's love for man and how that love/grace changes or impacts a person's life for good. Continue to allow His grace to change you.

Prayer: God, thank you for your grace and how it has and will continue to change me.

Journal Your Journey: In what ways has God's grace changed you?

ME < GOD

Journal Your Journey:

Track Your Day - Date: _____/_____/_____

Breakfast	Snack	Lunch	Snack	Dinner	Snack

Water Intake:

Exercise:

Day 70 – Train Your Body

I discipline my body like an athlete, training it to do what it should. Otherwise, I fear that after preaching to others I myself might be disqualified. 1 Corinthians 9:27 NLT

I am blessed to have a husband that takes good care of me and does kind things like open my car door, and dropping me off under an awning when it is raining and then goes to park the car. He had also gotten in the habit of dropping me off if we had to park some distance from where we were entering a building, so I didn't have to walk. This was him being a gentleman and partially because of me, being overweight with no energy to walk.

I feel better, energy-wise, than I've felt since being a teenager. I realize now how much being overweight impacted my energy and desire to be active because it was just plain tiring, I don't ever want to feel that way again. Exercise has become a natural and daily part of my life. If I don't do it, I miss it. Because it was a habit for my husband to drop me off, so I didn't have to walk, I have to remind him now as he pulls up to a door that I'll walk with him and he can park anywhere he'd like.

Our bodies are God's temple. He desires for us to train and discipline our bodies and to take care of them. Our bodies were created for movement, not to be sedentary. Research shows that lack of movement causes many health risks and concerns. I know it takes time and effort to exercise, but the rewards are so great. My friend, if you are not physically active, start now, start small. If you are already active, encourage those around you who aren't active by inviting them to do things with you.

Prayer: God, thank you for a body that moves and functions the way you created it to.

Journal Your Journey: Are you training and disciplining your body?

ME < GOD

Journal Your Journey:

Track Your Day - Date: _____/_____/_____

Breakfast	Snack	Lunch	Snack	Dinner	Snack

Water Intake:

Exercise:

Day 71 – More Alike Than We Think

Then Peter replied, "I see very clearly that God shows no favoritism. In every nation he accepts those who fear him and do what is right. This is the message of Good News for the people of Israel—that there is peace with God through Jesus Christ, who is Lord of all. Acts 10:34-36 NLT

I recently met a woman at a health event. As she and I talked and were getting to know each other, I learned that she was born in Malaysia but grew up in Australia. I shared about my goal to lose 100 pounds and keep it off, and she told me about her goal to lose 8 pounds. She is a very petite woman, so these 8 pounds had been plaguing her for 5 years and had been difficult to lose. She said she had tried numerous things and they just wouldn't come off. But, she had just reached her goal using the same eating plan I've been using the past three months.

I recalled how I had plateaued earlier this year after losing 40 pounds but was not losing anymore and had struggled for 5 months at that weight. I realized that it doesn't matter whether you have 8 pounds or 100 pounds to lose, it is about being the healthiest and best version of yourself.

This is the amazing thing about our relationship with God; each of us is different, grew up in different cultures, struggle with different issues and have different goals, yet we are all the same in God's eyes. He loves us all the same, shows no favoritism or is no respecter of persons.

So, whatever your goal is my friend, know that God sees you, He knows when you struggle, He knows when you succeed, He loves you and cares about what you care about. That is good news!

Prayer: Thank you, God, for loving us all the same and at the same time caring about what we individually care about.

Journal Your Journey: Do you realize that no matter how small or how big your weight loss goal, God cares about it and you?

ME < GOD

Journal Your Journey:

Track Your Day - Date: _____/_____/_____

Breakfast	Snack	Lunch	Snack	Dinner	Snack

Water Intake:
▯ ▯ ▯ ▯ ▯ ▯

Exercise:

Day 72 – No Need to Compare Yourself

Pay careful attention to your own work, for then you will get the satisfaction of a job well done, and you won't need to compare yourself to anyone else. For we are each responsible for our own conduct. Galatians 6:4-5 NLT

I have been hesitant to engage in social media because there is a component of it that just vexes my soul. One reason is I am a Human Resources professional, and sometimes I look at what is posted by some people, and I want to coach them against posting such things because I know other people may judge them based on their posts.

But, what bothers me the most is the feeling of comparing yourself to others; what they have done or are doing. This may not be something that you deal with, but I have dealt with the negative spirit of comparison. It is such a trap that lures you in because you haven't accomplished the things you desire, because of low self-esteem, because of what someone has said to you, or better yet because of what you have said to yourself.

A wise friend once cautioned me against comparing myself to others, and she said, "When you compare yourself to others you always come up short or feeling superior, and either way, it is untrue." We all are worthy, valuable, and deserve respect and dignity. Having hundreds of followers or being famous doesn't make you better than another person. But, this crazy world we live in, particularly on social media, can cause you to think that is what is relevant or real.

Of course, there are many positive things I see posted as well and if this is a tool you use positively, keep it up, my friend; we need more positivity in social media.

Prayer: God, thank you that you don't, and I don't have to, compare myself to anyone or anything except your word and your will for my life.

Journal Your Journey: Have you compared yourself to others and felt either superior or less than them?

ME < GOD

Journal Your Journey:

Track Your Day - Date: _____/_____/_____

Breakfast	Snack	Lunch	Snack	Dinner	Snack

Water Intake:
⊔ ⊔ ⊔ ⊔ ⊔ ⊔ ⊔

Exercise:

Day 73 – Healing The Brokenhearted

He heals the brokenhearted And binds up their wounds [healing their pain and comforting their sorrow]. Psalm 147:3 AMP

Do you ever wonder why bad things happen to innocent people? Such as the molestation of children, sex trafficking of girls and women, or when people take advantage of a person's kindness or generosity. A typical reaction in these situations is for the victim to blame themselves and to feel condemnation, which is a tactic the enemy uses against us.

When these types of violations occur, it can cause the victim to turn to destructive habits such as drugs, alcohol, promiscuity, or overeating; sometimes all of these, to escape the pain of the situation. A friend of mine wrote a book about her journey. It is called, "Releasing the Weight of My Past." She shared how when she started writing the book it was only going to be about her weight loss journey, but God used her and her suffering to bring healing to herself and many other women.

When bad things happen to innocent people, it is not God that is causing it, it is people. Our loving God has given us all the freedom to choose. He desires that we would choose Him, and learn to be like Him, but not everyone does; so bad things happen to innocent people by other people. Also, God does not promise that we won't have suffering or that we'll have a perfect life when we choose Him, but what He does promise is a perfect eternity and peace in the midst of pain or suffering.

My friend, if your weight loss journey has involved the pain you endured at the hands of another person, know that it is not your fault and that you are not alone. God is a healer, and He is able to heal us of everything.

Prayer: Thank you, God, for healing me, especially in places that I didn't even know needed healing.

Journal Your Journey: Have you endured pain at the hands of another person? If so, acknowledge that it is not your fault. Write in your journal "X happened to me, but it is not my fault."

ME < GOD

Journal Your Journey:

Track Your Day - Date: _____/_____/_____

Breakfast	Snack	Lunch	Snack	Dinner	Snack

Water Intake:
⊔ ⊔ ⊔ ⊔ ⊔ ⊔

Exercise:

Day 74 – Hope & Encouragement

Why am I discouraged? Why is my heart so sad? I will put my hope in God! I will praise him again— my Savior and my God! Psalm 43:5 NLT

I had a doctor's appointment recently that was disappointing for me. My first visit to this doctor was just over a year ago, and she informed me that my A1C level was in the pre-diabetic range and that I needed to lose weight and change my eating habits or I'd be heading towards having Type II Diabetes. She prescribed Metformin for me to take and recommended I lose weight.

According to their scale (of course mine is better because I don't have on clothes and shoes!), I've lost 55 pounds since I started seeing her, and now my A1C is in the normal range. But, she recommended I continue to take Metformin until I reach my goal of losing 100 pounds. That was not what I wanted to hear, because I hate swallowing pills.

But, I was also disappointed because her reaction to me losing 55 pounds was less than exciting. I don't know what I was expecting, but I didn't get it. I set a personal goal to lose 100 pounds that was not what she suggested, she just said to lose some weight. So, I guess I at least expected her to be happy for me, excited, encouraging, or to have some sort of celebratory tone. Nothing?

Whether other people celebrate you, recognize what you've done, or acknowledge it, it is crucial to lose weight for your own personal reasons, so that no matter what other people do or don't do, it doesn't hinder you from reaching your goal. God is always there to encourage you, support you and celebrate with you. Our relationship with Him gives us hope that empowers us to face every disappointment.

Prayer: God, thank you for helping me through disappointment and for reminding me that I always have hope and encouragement through you.

Journal Your Journey: Have you been disappointed by someone's reaction to your weight loss?

ME < GOD

Journal Your Journey:

Track Your Day - Date: _____/_____/_____

Breakfast	Snack	Lunch	Snack	Dinner	Snack

Water Intake:

Exercise:

Day 75 – Who Told You That?

"Who told you that you were naked?" the Lord God asked. "Have you eaten from the tree whose fruit I commanded you not to eat?" Genesis 3:11 NLT

I recently become aware of the terms body image and body image advocates. This wasn't something I'd heard of growing up even though it impacted my life. It is said the phrase body image was coined in 1935 by psychoanalyst, Paul Schilder. Body image was a concern in the Garden of Eden and has been ever since.

Body image can be defined as how one views themselves in the mirror or in their mind. Our society places a high value on beauty according to its standards, and some people believe that their body doesn't measure up to these standards. This causes shame, self-consciousness, and to feel like others are more attractive.

Dove's Choose Beautiful commercial where women all over the world were given the option to walk through one of two doors; one labeled beautiful and the other labeled average, was compelling to watch because many women chose the average door. Some talked about how they later regretted that they decided to walk through that door versus the beautiful door because they rated themselves, it wasn't someone else rating them.

My friend, if you have struggled with your body image, you are not alone. I have and other women have too. A couple of ways to overcome body image issues is truth and gratitude. The truth, or what God says about your body versus your negative thoughts or words. He says your body is His temple, and it is fearfully and wonderfully made. As well as, being grateful for a body that moves and functions the way God created it.

Prayer: God, thank you for the truth of your word. I will refuse to listen to or believe lies about my body.

Journal Your Journey: Have you struggled with your body image?

ME < GOD

Journal Your Journey:

Track Your Day - Date: _____/_____/_____

Breakfast	Snack	Lunch	Snack	Dinner	Snack

Water Intake:

Exercise:

Day 76 – Nothing New Under The Sun

History merely repeats itself. It has all been done before. Nothing under the sun is truly new. Ecclésiastes 1:9 NLT

Even though there are thousands of diet or weight loss products on the market and the weight loss industry is estimated to be worth $68.2 billion in 2017, there still is only one thing that causes weight loss over time; taking in fewer calories than you expend. I know, it sounds simple, and I understand, believe me, that it is not easy.

There really is nothing truly new under the sun. So, the latest this or that may or may not be the answer you are seeking on your weight loss journey. What I do know for sure is that you have to decide what you are going to do and then stick to that. God will lead and guide you to what is right for you and your body. As you continue to seek Him daily and give your weight loss to Him, He will do more than you can ask or think.

Prayer: God, thank you for leading me to the right weight loss regimen for me, and that I am consistent with that plan.

Journal Your Journey: Have you decided what you are going to do to lose weight and keep it off? Are you sticking to that plan?

ME < GOD

Journal Your Journey:

Track Your Day - Date: _____ / _____ / _____

Breakfast	Snack	Lunch	Snack	Dinner	Snack

Water Intake:
☐ ☐ ☐ ☐ ☐ ☐ ☐

Exercise:

Day 77 – One Race

Then the Lord God formed the man from the dust of the ground. He breathed the breath of life into the man's nostrils, and the man became a living person. Genesis 2:7 NLT

I attended a remarkable event, the OneRace Movement, at Stone Mountain. It was an event to promote racial healing, and that celebrated the 55th anniversary of Dr. Martin Luther King Jr.'s "I Have A Dream" speech: "Let freedom ring from Stone Mountain of Georgia." The event brought together leaders of all races and ethnicities from across the region, and thousands of people stood together in unity on the vast lawn of Stone Mountain Park, renouncing the spirit of racism. It was powerful!

I was also excited about how I felt physically. This was my first time at Stone Mountain. The park has a lot of uneven terrains and requires a lot of walking. I felt great and had lots of energy as my friends, and I walked throughout the park. This would not have been the case 55 pounds ago! I would have been exhausted and in pain.

Losing weight is so much more than looking good in our clothes. The physical aspect of weight loss allows you to be active and to have more energy, which causes you to have a richer and more fulfilling life. God created us to move. He breathed life into Adam, from which we all descended, one race. He created all of us to be physically active beings, not sedentary. So be active my friend, and enjoy the body God has given you.

Prayer: Thank you, God, that we are one race, your people, and thank you for giving me the ability to be physically active.

Journal Your Journey: What unexpected things have happened to you as a result of your weight loss, that have made your life richer and fuller?

ME < GOD

Journal Your Journey:

Track Your Day - Date: _____/_____/_____

Breakfast	Snack	Lunch	Snack	Dinner	Snack

Water Intake:

Exercise:

Day 78 – Promises

Do not be afraid or discouraged, for the Lord will personally go ahead of you. He will be with you; he will neither fail you nor abandon you."
Deuteronomy 31:8 NLT

Has someone ever promised to do something for you and didn't keep their promise? Have you ever found it easier to keep a promise to someone else more so than keeping one with yourself? Have you broken a promise to others or to God? Unfortunately, I have done all three.

Each time we break a promise to ourselves, it impacts our confidence. It can be a self-defeating cycle. Many times we may make a promise to ourselves, but don't have a plan or strategy as to how we were going to accomplish what we intended to do, so we were bound to fail. The good news is that you can stop this cycle and begin to make and keep promises to yourself.

God does not condemn us, so forgive yourself for broken promises and ask God to help you make the right promises and to keep them. In this passage of scripture, Moses was telling Joshua what God would do through him and God's promises. God's promises are sure and you can always count on them and Him.

Prayer: God, help me to make the right promises and to keep them, especially to myself.

Journal Your Journey: What promises have you broken to yourself?

ME < GOD

Journal Your Journey:

Track Your Day - Date: _____/_____/_____

Breakfast	Snack	Lunch	Snack	Dinner	Snack

Water Intake:
🥛 🥛 🥛 🥛 🥛 🥛 🥛

Exercise:

Day 79 – Advisers & Accountability

So don't go to war without wise guidance; victory depends on having many advisers. Proverbs 24:6 NLT

Pride and offense are two of Satan's best strategies because most of us fall for them the majority of the time unless we learn to recognize them and not allow them to entrap us. When you are working towards losing weight, pride and offense can definitely come in and trap you. I tell you this from experience, my friend.

My husband and I will celebrate 12 years of marriage this year. In those 12 years, I've struggled to lose weight, and my weight has yo-yoed up and down. My husband has been understanding and supportive the majority of the time, but despite that, I have been offended and prideful many times.

This may sound familiar to you. I have told my husband that I am on a specific eating plan or not eating something, then my husband would see me doing the opposite of what I said and would say something to me about what I told him. He knows how much I want to lose weight, so he tries to help me and remind me of what I told him. How do you think I have responded most times? You guessed it, with strife or anger, because I was offended.

My friend, you may have a loved one, a friend, or a coach, that you have shared your sincere desire to lose weight with. There is wisdom in having advisers and accountability. Out of love and concern for you, they may have brought you in remembrance of what you said or tried to advise you. Don't allow offense or pride to cause you to get stuck in a place where it hinders your weight loss or your relationships. Recognize it for what it is, apologize for your behavior and part in the offense and move forward towards your goal.

Prayer: God, thank you for revealing to me when I am offended and to forgive myself, apologize to those I need to apologize to and move forward.

Journal Your Journey: Have you been offended or prideful during your weight loss journey?

ME < GOD

Journal Your Journey:

Track Your Day - Date: _____/_____/_____

Breakfast	Snack	Lunch	Snack	Dinner	Snack

Water Intake:
◯ ◯ ◯ ◯ ◯ ◯ ◯

Exercise:

Day 80 – You Will Be Tempted

And don't let us yield to temptation, but rescue us from the evil one.
Matthew 6:13 NLT

My Dad used to call me Junk Food Junkie because I would want to eat junk food more than any other food. My eating habits were poor for years. As I've gotten older, I've increased my palate and improved my eating habits, but there have been many times where I have merely craved all the wrong things.

When I was on vacation, visiting with my husband's family in Rochester, NY, it was the first time in months that I was tempted to eat something, not on my eating plan. But, by the grace of God, I resisted temptation. How I did it was by thinking about my goal and asking God to help me in my weakness.

Today's scripture is from the passage of scriptures where God is teaching us about how to pray and fast. Apparently, we will have temptation, as He doesn't tell us to pray to remove temptation from us. Instead, He tells us to pray to not yield to temptation. So my friend, know that you will be tempted on this journey, but that God is able to help you not yield to temptation.

Prayer: God, thank you for keeping me from yielding to temptation.

Journal Your Journey: How will you handle temptation?

ME < GOD

Journal Your Journey:

Track Your Day - Date: _____/_____/_____

Breakfast	Snack	Lunch	Snack	Dinner	Snack

Water Intake:
▢ ▢ ▢ ▢ ▢ ▢ ▢

Exercise:

Day 81 — He Sees You

Thereafter, Hagar used another name to refer to the Lord, who had spoken to her. She said, "You are the God who sees me." She also said, "Have I truly seen the One who sees me?" Genesis 16:13 NLT

Have there been times that you found yourself doing things that you knew you shouldn't have done and then you tried to hide it from others and even tried to hide it from yourself? I have, I have eaten things I knew I shouldn't have and did it while I was in the car driving home to or from work, so my husband wouldn't know and hold me accountable like I asked him to. Then I've been disappointed or even surprised when I didn't get the results I wanted.

If you have done something similar, my friend, you are not alone. God sees us and knows everything we do and don't do. He will correct us, comfort us, coach us and console us. Hagar had run away from her master, Sarai because she had done something she should not have done to Sarai; and Sarai then treated her harshly, so Hagar ran away. But, it didn't matter where she tried to hide, God saw her and knew all that had taken place. He didn't love her any less because of what she had done. He comforted her and coached her to go back to Sarai. God does the same with us. No matter what we do, He won't love us any less. He is the God who sees us, so there is no need to hide what we've done from Him.

Prayer: God, thank you for seeing me and loving me no matter what.

Journal Your Journey: Have there been times that you found yourself doing things that you knew you shouldn't have done and then you tried to hide it from others and even tried to hide it from yourself?

ME < GOD

Journal Your Journey:

Track Your Day - Date: _____/_____/_____

Breakfast	Snack	Lunch	Snack	Dinner	Snack

Water Intake:
◯ ◯ ◯ ◯ ◯ ◯ ◯

Exercise:

Day 82 – Infinitely More Than We Think

Now all glory to God, who is able, through his mighty power at work within us, to accomplish infinitely more than we might ask or think. Ephesians 3:20 NLT

The last time I spent time with our nieces and nephew in Rochester, NY, we went to a trampoline park, and I decided to jump in a foam ball pit with one of the younger ones, and I couldn't get out! I struggled to pull myself up out of those foam balls, and I would sink like a bag of potatoes in quicksand. My weight and lack of abdominal strength prohibited me from being able to get out on my own. A 16-year old that worked there had to get down in the foam pit with me and help me out.

This year it has been entirely different. I've been able to do everything with the kids that they want to do and I am not limited because of my weight. When I set out to lose 100 pounds and to keep it off, this was not one of the reasons I thought of as one of my "whys" to lose weight. But, now that I have lost weight, it feels great to have this as a by-product; able to play freely with my nieces and nephew. God is amazing, and He will do more than we might ask or think.

Prayer: God, thank you for doing more than what I asked for or thought of. Thank you for all of the many benefits of weight loss.

Journal Your Journey: What has God done that is more than you asked or thought of when you started your weight loss journey?

ME < GOD

Journal Your Journey:

Track Your Day - Date: _____/_____/_____

Breakfast	Snack	Lunch	Snack	Dinner	Snack

Water Intake: ⌢⌢⌢⌢⌢⌢⌢

Exercise:

Day 83 – The Secret

I know how to live on almost nothing or with everything. I have learned the secret of living in every situation, whether it is with a full stomach or empty, with plenty or little.
Philippians 4:12 NLT

My Pastor used to demonstrate how frustration manifests by drawing imaginary lines in the air, one higher than the other; the highest line is what you expected, and the lower line is what actually occurred. He'd say that frustration is all of the space in between the two lines. Naturally, we have high expectations sometimes for our family and friends.

But, there are times when you hope that your family or friends will react or behave like you expect or want them to; and when that doesn't happen, it can be frustrating. In these types of situations, it can cause you to act out in ways that you don't want, such as overeating; or what is called emotional eating.

Of course, emotionally eating is a temporary fix and doesn't resolve the situation you are dealing with; since the issue will still be there after you finish eating. So, how do you stop emotional eating? Experts provide many different techniques, and many of them start with acknowledging what or how you are feeling and then being mindful of what you are eating. I agree with these techniques, and I know that learning the secret of living in every situation, being content in every situation, as the Apostle Paul writes in Philippians is also a good strategy.

Prayer: God, thank you for helping me to be content in every situation.

Journal Your Journey: Have you learned the secret?

ME < GOD

Journal Your Journey:

Track Your Day - Date: _____/_____/_____

Breakfast	Snack	Lunch	Snack	Dinner	Snack

Water Intake:

Exercise:

Day 84 – Accept Yourself & Others

In this new life, it doesn't matter if you are a Jew or a Gentile, circumcised or uncircumcised, barbaric, uncivilized, slave, or free. Christ is all that matters, and he lives in all of us. Colossians 3:11 NLT

There are many ways we are different as human beings, our culture, upbringing, how we handle conflict, and of course the most obvious our skin tone. But there are many ways we are alike as well; such as our desire to be loved, respected and accepted.

Everyone wants to be accepted for who they are, and there is nothing worse than feeling like you have to change to be accepted by others or feeling like others believe they are better than you. But as one of my favorite quotes by Eleanor Roosevelt says, 'No one can make you feel inferior without your consent.' Regardless of what people say, do or think, you have to know who you are.

God created all of us, and He created us all different for a reason. If you don't like the differences that God placed in you, then you are telling God He made a mistake when He created you, and that is not possible. So, come to terms with the uniqueness of who God created you to be and accept others for who God created them to be.

Prayer: God, thank you for making all of us different, yet the same in your eyes. I accept exactly who you made me to be and I accept others as they are.

Journal Your Journey: What things about yourself do you still need to accept?

ME < GOD

Journal Your Journey:

Track Your Day - Date: _____/_____/_____

Breakfast	Snack	Lunch	Snack	Dinner	Snack

Water Intake:

Exercise:

Day 85 – God Gives You The Power

Remember the Lord your God. He is the one who gives you power to be successful, in order to fulfill the covenant he confirmed to your ancestors with an oath. Deuteronomy 8:18 NLT

A legendary icon, Aretha Franklin, was laid to rest recently. The world watched as she was honored and eulogized. A few times I heard news reporters give a summary of her life as they were introducing a segment about her, and they would mention how she struggled with her weight at times in her life.

It is interesting how this was a part of the summary of her life, but her struggle with weight never hindered her from being the 'Queen of Soul' and a legendary icon around the world. There is a lesson to be learned from this; regardless of what you struggle with, it should not stop you from doing what God has called you to do; or specifically, that struggling with weight does not prohibit you from being highly successful and respected by many in a competitive industry. This means you too can be successful regardless of your weight. Remember that our prosperity and success comes from God.

Prayer: God, thank you for making me successful.

Journal Your Journey: Are you allowing your weight to keep you from being successful?

ME < GOD

Journal Your Journey:

Track Your Day - Date: _____/_____/_____

Breakfast	Snack	Lunch	Snack	Dinner	Snack

Water Intake:

Exercise:

Day 86 – Put On Your New Nature

Put on your new nature, and be renewed as you learn to know your Creator and become like him. Colossians 3:10 NLT

There are a few schools of thought when it comes to eating. One thought is that I eat to live, not for enjoyment. Another is that I eat for enjoyment or pleasure, not to live. And, yet another thought is that I eat to live and for pleasure. I prefer the latter. I want to eat for energy and for enjoyment, and it is possible to eat healthily and enjoy what you eat.

Sometimes there are things we eat, and even though it may have tasted good, we feel sluggish and regret eating it. When it comes to losing weight, we have to learn to adjust our palate and explore alternatives to what we may have eaten in the past that is not good for us. After a period of time, you'll find that you have adjusted your eating habits and that you don't even miss those things that weren't good for you.

Our life in Christ is similar in that we learn to be like Him every day. You learn to enjoy the goodness of God in everything. At first, it seems foreign to act or respond differently, as we put off our old nature or behaviors. But after a while, it becomes natural to respond with love in every situation. Even when the other person may be wrong and you want to respond the way you have in the past with anger, sarcasm, or snidely. God renews your thinking and your behavior changes because you have put on your new nature.

Prayer: God, thank you that I am becoming more like you. Thank you for my new nature, that desires to eat healthily.

Journal Your Journey: Recall a time when you realized that you responded differently (more like Christ) than you had in the past.

ME < GOD

Journal Your Journey:

Track Your Day - Date: _____/_____/_____

Breakfast	Snack	Lunch	Snack	Dinner	Snack

Water Intake:

Exercise:

Day 87 – We All Struggle at Times

Live creatively, friends. If someone falls into sin, forgivingly restore him, saving your critical comments for yourself. You might be needing forgiveness before the days out. Stoop down and reach out to those who are oppressed. Share their burdens, and so complete Christ's law. If you think you are too good for that, you are badly deceived. Galatians 6:1 MSG

I read a post today of a woman sharing about her struggle to stay focused on her eating plan while she traveled for vacation. She said she didn't eat right the whole time she was on her trip and now that she was back at home, she regretted it and was trying to get back on track. I could relate to her pain because I have been there.

It is like the saying goes, you take one step forward and two steps back; which means you end up in a worse situation then when you started. You not only lose ground on your journey towards your goals, you potentially gain weight, feel regret, disappointment, and frustration. But, once it is done, there is nothing you can do to change the past. You have to focus on the future, forgive yourself, and determine what you will do if that situation comes up again.

God wants us to support and encourage each other, so learn to reach out to those who will support you during those times that you feel tempted to take two steps back. We all struggle at times, be there to encourage others and others will be there to encourage you.

Prayer: God, thank you for showing me how to support others and how to seek and receive support when I need it.

Journal Your Journey: Who will you reach out to for support when you feel tempted?

ME < GOD

Journal Your Journey:

Track Your Day - Date: _____/_____/_____

Breakfast	Snack	Lunch	Snack	Dinner	Snack

Water Intake: ⌒ ⌒ ⌒ ⌒ ⌒ ⌒ ⌒

Exercise:

Day 88 – Your Journey

Then they said, "Ask God whether or not our journey will be successful." "Go in peace," the priest replied. "For the Lord is watching over your journey." Judges 18:5-6 NLT

Journey is both a noun and a verb. As a noun, the dictionary defines it as an act of traveling from one place to another. As a verb, it is described as to travel somewhere. This weight loss journey is definitely both.

Sometimes you are merely traveling somewhere; to that next pound or milestone, you are trying to reach. Then there is your overall journey, you aren't sure when you'll achieve your goal, but you physically start at one weight (place), and you hope to travel to a lower weight (place). Throughout your journey, there will be valleys, peaks, rough and smooth terrain that you will go through. You have to go through it. No one else can take this journey for you, as everyone's journey is different. But, rest assured my friend, that God is watching over your journey.

Prayer: God, thank you for my journey and for being with me every step of the way.

Journal Your Journey: Have you officially asked God to be with you during every step of your weight loss journey?

ME < GOD

Journal Your Journey:

Track Your Day - Date: _____/_____/_____

Breakfast	Snack	Lunch	Snack	Dinner	Snack

Water Intake: ☐ ☐ ☐ ☐ ☐ ☐

Exercise:

Day 89 – Working Together For The Good

And we know that God causes everything to work together for the good of those who love God and are called according to his purpose for them.
Romans 8:28 NLT

Life doesn't always go as we plan. We may have thought or hoped we'd be further along in our weight loss journey than where we are now. The timing we had in mind as to when we'd lose the weight, may not be the time frame in which it happens. But, I can assure you, my friend, if you remain consistent it will happen in God's timing.

Romans 8:28 has always brought me comfort, because even when things don't go as I've planned, even though I may be disappointed, frustrated, and questioning why, inevitably things always work together for good. I may not see or understand that at the time something doesn't go my way, but in time, I see it and thank God for His love and protection, as I am reminded of this promise.

I pray that you too find comfort in His word that He causes everything to work together for good. When things haven't gone your way, text yourself this scripture; or write it on a Post-It Note and put it on your walls or mirrors, so that you can find peace and joy in the midst of that situation.

Prayer: God, thank you that even when I don't lose the weight I had hoped in the timeframe I was hoping, I know that it will happen in your timing if I stay focused because you work all things together for good.

Journal Your Journey: Write or copy this scripture, Romans 8:28, in your journal and reflect on it by capturing your feelings and thoughts in writing.

ME < GOD

Journal Your Journey:

Track Your Day - Date: _____/_____/_____

Breakfast	Snack	Lunch	Snack	Dinner	Snack

Water Intake:

Exercise:

Day 90 – More Than Words…Well-Made Weapons

And that about wraps it up. God is strong, and he wants you strong. So take everything the Master has set out for you, well-made weapons of the best materials. And put them to use so you will be able to stand up to everything the Devil throws your way. This is no afternoon athletic contest that we'll walk away from and forget about in a couple of hours. This is for keeps, a life-or-death fight to the finish against the Devil and all his angels. Be prepared. You're up against far more than you can handle on your own. Take all the help you can get, every weapon God has issued, so that when it's all over but the shouting you'll still be on your feet. Truth, righteousness, peace, faith, and salvation are more than words. Learn how to apply them. You'll need them throughout your life. God's Word is an indispensable weapon. In the same way, prayer is essential in this ongoing warfare. Pray hard and long. Pray for your brothers and sisters. Keep your eyes open. Keep each other's spirits up so that no one falls behind or drops out. And don't forget to pray for me. Pray that I'll know what to say and have the courage to say it at the right time, Ephesians 6:10-19 MSG

Well, my friend, we have come to the end of this leg of our journey together. I pray that you have found there is less of you and more of God in your life and that He is leading and guiding you more than ever.

We end our time together with a passage of scripture that sums up the best way to make it through this journey, and that will give you the strength you need to finish. As it says, truth, righteousness, peace, faith, and salvation are more than words; learn how to apply them; you'll need them throughout your life. So how do we apply them?

Truth - God's word is true and is what we can rely on in every situation. There indeed is a word for every situation you may face, even for your weight loss journey as you have hopefully learned. If you aren't sure what word to apply to your situation, use study Bibles, commentaries, Pastors, fellow believers, but most importantly ask God to help you understand His word and His truth.

Righteousness - God calls us righteous or justified, which means as His child and through His grace we have been made right, free from all sin, such as deceit, pride, lust, stealing, covetousness, or jealousy. This doesn't mean we won't be tempted by our old nature to sin, but if we do, He gives us the ability to repent and get right back to being justified. Applying this is essential so that you don't condemn yourself and allow guilt to keep you in that state.

Peace - there is nothing like the peace of God. His peace allows us to be at peace in the midst of any situation. The world is not able to give this type of peace. It is actually designed to steal our peace and cause anxiety, fear, and confusion. Apply peace by spending time in God's presence on a regular basis, and He will keep you in perfect peace.

Faith - the word of God says that faith is the substance of things hoped for and the evidence of things not seen, Faith in God, who He is, what He did for us to save us, and what He does for us each day takes faith. Because it isn't something you can see, but it is something you must believe to receive. If you believe, you know that you can trust God's wisdom, guidance, provision, and protection in every situation.

Salvation - in its purest form, salvation means that God sent Jesus Christ to rescue us from the many consequences of our sin. Once you accept Jesus Christ as your Lord and Savior, you are saved. God, then begins to mold and shape you into being more and more like Him which is a daily process. To grow into full spiritual maturity, you have to consistently study God's word, following His commands and receiving His guidance.

These are powerful weapons that God has given you to succeed in life, and that includes in your weight loss journey. Use them as often as possible and share them with others so they may have success too.

I am excited to hear what God has done in your life and the results that have manifested on your weight loss journey. Remember I am on this journey with you my friend, so I will continue to pray for you, and I ask that you pray for me as well. Until we meet again, be good to others and to yourself.

Prayer: God, thank you for my weapons that I can use throughout my life for every situation, and especially right now God on my weight loss journey.

Journal Your Journey: Whether you've reached your goal weight or not, what is your plan to continue this journey or to keep the weight off?

ME < GOD

Journal Your Journey:

Track Your Day - Date: _____/_____/_____

Breakfast	Snack	Lunch	Snack	Dinner	Snack

Water Intake:
🥛 🥛 🥛 🥛 🥛 🥛 🥛

Exercise:

About the Author

Leslie Baldwin is a human resources professional, facilitator, trainer, mediator, and most importantly, woman of God. She desires to add value to other people's lives through personal examples of her own life, teaching, encouraging and helping other people succeed. Her prayer is that others realize they are not alone and that God loves them deeply.

Leslie is married to Nelson E. Baldwin Jr. and they live in Alpharetta, GA where they both serve in marketplace ministry and enjoy spending time with their family, especially their beautiful granddaughter, Ana.

To get in touch with Leslie, to share your testimony, how this book has blessed you, or for speaking engagements, you can contact her at:

Repairers of the Breach Consulting, LLC
PO Box 5462
Alpharetta, GA 30023
Phone: 706-580-6035
Email: lesliertbsolutions@gmail.com

Made in the USA
Middletown, DE
22 December 2018